"TRUST ME, I'M A DOCTOR"

Understanding and Surviving Modern Health Care

Thomas L. Minogue, M.D.

TLM Consulting &
Medical Communications

Acknowledgments

I would like to thank those who made a contribution to this book. These people are far too numerous to mention by name and include many, many family members and friends. However, particular note should be made of the following who read and commented on the manuscript:

Sari Aronson, M.D.; Laurie Gibbons;
Benjamin H. Levi, M.D., Ph.D.; & Martha Schaafsma, RN.

ISBN 0-9654891-0-8

Printed in the United States of America
Design by Stephen Kirby

TLM Consulting, P.O. Box 293,
Monticello, Illinois 61856-0293

Medical Communications, P. O. Box 954,
Urbana, Illinois 61801

To Pat

Table of Contents

Part One: Looking Behind the "Sterile Curtain"

Part Two: Getting Better Care

Part Three: Prognosis

Appendices

Preface

The *essentials* of good health care will never change; the *way* that care is delivered is constantly changing.

This book was written for those who would like to better understand the delivery of their own care—and the nation's health needs. It is for those who feel powerless or uninformed before a system that appears chaotic, complex, and virtually unknowable. It is for those who would take ultimate responsibility for their own medical destinies in a rapidly changing—and sometimes hostile—medical world.

Yes, various governmental and health industry designs for our care may be developing rapidly even as this book goes to press. Over the next few years those changes are likely to focus on finances more than on the care per se. In such a swiftly evolving system, people will more than ever need the kind of understanding that "*Trust Me, I'm a Doctor*" attempts to provide.

I wrote this book because I strongly believe that my unique experiences can help you understand and take more control of your health care.

To help accomplish these goals, I'll use an approach learned when I was a medical student. My teachers often had certain pieces of clinical knowledge which they thought were *especially* important for the students to know. They would dispense these to us as "clinical pearls"—small, discrete, focused chunks of information or even wisdom. I'll try to do much the same for you. At the beginning of each chapter (or at the beginning of each section, in the case of Chapter Twenty), you'll find a "pearl" to help focus you on an important message within it.

I'm also introducing the terms "Business-Medical Complex" and "Biz-Med Complex." To my knowledge this represents the first use of these in print. They'll be defined in Chapter One. Should the reader be aware of any earlier use, I would be grateful to be so informed. Credit can then be given as reasonable opportunity presents itself.

It's my fervent hope that you find *"Trust Me, I'm a Doctor"* to be interesting, innovative, but mostly helpful in your care.

Caution

Material in this book addresses many complex concerns people have about their health care. My comments are presented only as general considerations toward the goal of improving mental and physical well-being. As such, they are not a substitute for a personal, quality, patient-doctor relationship. No specific clinical application to any particular situation is implied or intended. Serious medical decisions should be made only after a careful evaluation of all relevant factors—along with the personal assistance of a competent practitioner.

Information provided in this book should not be read in isolation, but rather within the context of the entire work. I acknowledge many comments are generalizations, not true of all organizations or participants or applicable in all situations. Additionally, no endorsement is either intended or implied regarding any facility or organization mentioned within this book. They are cited for the purposes of illustration or as sources for further information. Finally, this book is by no means all-inclusive. While it tries to cover as much material as possible, it also leaves out more than I would wish.

Regardless of its limitations, the author hopes that it adequately serves those readers who use it well.

—Thomas L. Minogue, M.D.

PART 1

Looking Behind the "Sterile Curtain"

CHAPTER 1

"If the patients only knew..." An Introduction

Pearl:
Most people have more control over their health care than they realize.

Confronting the Chaos

Americans have some of the best health care in the world. We also have some of the worst.

On the same day and in the same hospital or clinic, the quality of services delivered can range from superb to barely adequate or even fatal. Such hit-and-miss results can seem beyond comprehension. They aren't. You don't have to be a doctor to either understand the tragedies or to use the strengths of the system on your own behalf.

In this book, I hope to provide you with answers I have learned from my own 30-year career as a physician. My career has been nothing if not diverse and instructive. It has included family practice, surgery, emergency room care, psychiatry, clinical teaching, and medical administration. I've witnessed all extremes of care: from life-saving to life-ending—and almost everything in between.

Although I look back on my own practice mostly with pride, I also have regrets. Sometimes I have been as much a part of the problem as the solution. At least the view from so many perspectives has helped me to more realistically see the medical world and myself.

No doubt you've had your own glimpses of health care. A friend may tell you that Uncle Henry was a new man following his bypass surgery. However, she may also relate how her mom died after a doctor didn't give serious consideration to the complaint of a breast lump. Physicians at a trauma center will be credited with helping your neighbor survive a near-fatal auto accident. Meanwhile, a co-worker, who was otherwise the picture of good health, died during a routine "minor" surgery at the local community hospital.

What order can the opinions and advice of "experts" such as myself bring to such chaos? True, we can tell you how to take care of your diabetes or depression, your hernia or your cancer. However, there remains a literally critical issue about which physicians rarely teach the public: *Why* the system works the way it does—poorly and well—and *how* you can use that knowledge to help yourself and your family. Don't physicians have a responsibility to do that? Having information on the *process* of health care can be more important than having purely *clinical* information.

The process of care is what I intend to focus on in this book. This isn't information from the latest medical journals or scientific seminars. It's what I learned at the bedside, in the operating room and the office exam room. It's not statistics and formal research results. That sort of information is readily available in hundreds of books and articles—and some of it may even be correct. This is the *whys* and *hows* as I've lived them. It's my "physician-ly," but still imperfect, account to you. I'll do the best I can to turn my clinical experiences into your advantage during times of medical need.

As we go along, you might properly ask, "Is Dr. Minogue correct?" I can only respond that I'm reporting to you the best I can as I draw from a lifetime of medical experience. While I've only heard the saying "Trust me, I'm a doctor" used in jest, I hope you'll trust me enough to at least carefully consider many of the issues to be discussed in this book.

One important measure of validity is whether the information confirms your own experiences (first-hand or otherwise) in the doctor's office, the emergency room, the hospital, or even in the waiting room. Equally as important, regardless of whether or not you agree with me, are thoughts which might be stimulated in you on ways for more productive care.

Just because the medical world appears to be so complicated, don't despair of finding some simple solutions to your better care. As we look together behind the "sterile curtain" of the medical world, you'll get some basic knowledge and develop some reasonable approaches. With managed care further complicating matters, broad principles of understanding and clear plans of action will become increasingly necessary. Many patients will find that they can use these principles to make a vital difference. Or to paraphrase what one of my medical students recently taught *me*, "If the patients only knew that we don't hold their lives in our hands—they do!"

The Untapped Power of Patients

No one is likely to be a better manager of your care than you are. The ability to manage it effectively is within the reach of almost everyone. That's not to say it's an easy task.

In fact, my firm belief in patients' abilities underlies the basic premise of this book:

> Our most valuable untapped health care resource is *people*—their potential to understand how care is delivered, and to use that knowledge productively.

This statement applies to patients and caregivers alike.

We need to recognize that *understanding* and *empowerment* are the missing links to better personal care and to a more effective approach to national health care. Both of these links can—and must—become incorporated into the routine of our daily lives as much as money, sports, sex, or television; neither link should be reserved for only occasional use or crisis situations.

Without a workable understanding of the health care system, patients will be forever denied full participation in their own care. The personal results can be disastrous. But, if patients can acquire such useful knowledge, they can become more productive partners with their caregivers. In the best case scenario, this could take on the characteristics of a "collaborative practice" between them.

To focus on understanding and empowerment is not to deny other significant influences on the delivery of health care. Money, formal programs within the public and private sectors, skilled personnel, modern technology, and even "bricks and mortar" are among other important factors. But these are largely in place already, or are less central to the needed solutions, or have already fallen short of their promise. My emphasis in this book is on the more unrecognized and under-utilized resources of people's understanding and empowerment and the benefits which flow from them.

I want the approach I'm presenting to be as clear as possible. Briefly stated, understanding plus empowerment help lead to better care. Remember this progression:

UNDERSTANDING + EMPOWERMENT → BETTER CARE

Through understanding and empowerment, patients and providers can both bring about a major improvement in care.

In this quest for better care, there are basic questions to be answered. Here are some of the crucial ones: Is the purpose of health care as obvious as it seems? In day-to-day practice, how is that care really delivered? How can patients recognize when treatment may not be progressing satisfactorily? To what extent does the health care system interact with our larger society—and how does each change the other? How can patients more fully and actively participate in their own care? Is it truly in your best interest to have a delivery system based on primary care doctors? What is the role of the patient-doctor relationship in care? Where does the issue of *suffering* fit into this picture? Finally, how can the answers to these questions be put to use in practical, or even lifesaving, ways?

Part of a patient's task in achieving this can include the recognition of the very best and the very worst aspects of health care. An understanding of the influences which produce both extremes is then possible. This understanding helps bring empowerment to the patient as well as change to the system.

The Biz-Med Complex

To understand where you fit in today's health care, it helps to examine a bigger picture. The Business-Medical Complex, or "Biz-Med Complex," is the term I use for our country's extensive, interconnected system of medically related workers, services, organizations, and products. It's an expression analogous to "military-industrial complex." It also underscores the financial aspects involved in health care.

Medicine, dentistry, nursing and all the other healing professions which are part of the Complex should not be "businesses," although they do have financial components. And the remaining parts of the Biz-Med Complex, such as pharmaceutical and insurance companies, should never be only businesses.

The accompanying diagram (page 8) provides a simple graphic representation of the interaction of patients and the Biz-Med Complex. Currently, this Complex is at the *center* of the medical universe. Patients "revolve" around this Complex, with doctors as a part of its center, but not squarely so.

It shouldn't be this way. Patients should be at the center of the medical universe. The Biz-Med Complex should revolve around them. And doctors should be squarely at the core of the Complex.

The Medical Universe
Figure 1

O Biz-Med Complex   ◉ Doctors   ◎ Patients

The Way It Is

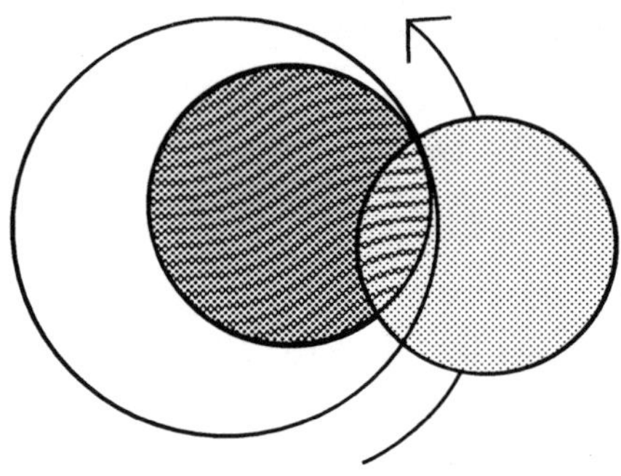

The Biz-Med Complex, with doctors skewed to the side, is currently at the center of this Universe. Patients now revolve around this complex.

. . .

The Way It Should Be

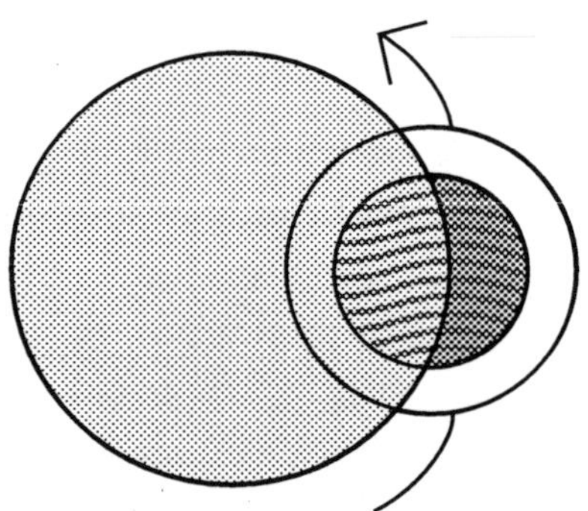

Patients should be at the center of this Universe, with the Biz-Med Complex revolving around them. Doctors should be squarely at the center of the Biz-Med Complex.

We'll examine ways to accomplish this as we progress through this book. Keep in mind that this Complex will become more "biz" and less "med" as managed care increases its share of the marketplace.

. . .

The Path Ahead

The best way to start your journey to the center of the medical universe is to have a good map, and a workable plan. For this, I offer you the "Four Steps to Better Care." They are:

1. *Understanding* ourselves, other people (including caregivers), our illnesses and the process of health care delivery.
2. *Involvement*—as actively and fully as possible—in disease prevention, early detection, and treatment; and in the relief of suffering generally.
3. *Responsibility* as an *obligation* to accept a personal role.
4. *Authority* as a *right* to be exercised in the interest of better care.

These "Four Steps to Better Care" can help you defeat a culture of helplessness, isolation, and inadequacy which is the fate of all too many patients—and, surprisingly, often the fate of doctors. These steps focus more on prevention than on treatment; they emphasize making smart decisions and avoiding unnecessary problems. While no completely "fail-safe" system exists in health care, patients can use the "Four Steps to Better Care" to work with physicians and other care providers to decrease potential risks. Providers can incorporate this approach into their work to enhance the care they give. The steps are so basic that they will be emphasized again and again in this book. They can help the entire system move toward a "culture of healing."

These steps are part of a larger process, that of empowerment. I like to imagine empowerment as having three components—its own ABCs.

The first component is Attitude. It's an "I-can-do-that" mindset that can come from a number of sources: idealism, necessity or frustration when confronted with illness, stimulation by consumer groups or political debate, being employed within the system, or even from the increased understanding and energy which a book such as this tries to engender. Any of these sources could provide the spark—the catalyst—necessary to overcome a feeling of powerlessness felt by many people.

The second component of empowerment is having a "Blueprint" which you can follow. It's pretty difficult to participate in something as complex as health care without an overall plan. For our purposes, the "Four Steps to Better Care" serve as the most basic blueprint.

Finally, a climate for Change helps to provide the fertile ground in which progress can occur. Of course, to make progress, it's necessary to *act* after empowerment. We'll talk more about these ABCs later.

. . .

The Doctor Is In

Much of this book focuses on the physician. It's important to understand him or her as a person, complete with everyday strengths and weaknesses. This helps the patient to recognize the doctor as approachable and within reach. Additionally, a more complete appreciation of the humanity of the physician can improve collaboration as well as offer additional protection from poor care.

To know the doctor is to know both the strongest and the weakest link in the chain of services and costs. To know the doctor is to know the very heart of the Biz-Med Complex. Yes, "the doctor is in" all right... right in the thick of it all.

The physician is seen as powerful, holding the cure for many of the physical and emotional problems of the patient. The structure of the entire Biz-Med Complex is built upon the relationship between patient and doctor.

Within the medical world, doctors have been unfairly maligned as well as unduly praised. They are simultaneously overvalued and undervalued, causing society even more confusion as it struggles with the true role of the physician. Regardless, the physician is crucial to the Biz-Med Complex, both controlling much of it and being controlled by it. To fail to understand the practitioner is to misunderstand the essential nature of health care.

In coming years, physicians will be further stressed to abide by the First Rule of Medicine: "Do no harm." And patients will need to take more responsibility in helping to prevent that harm to themselves.

To focus on doctors is not to ignore the triad of cost, quality, and access. These, too, will be addressed. But these ingredients are largely consequences flowing from physicians' thinking and actions.

When all the turf issues and political issues are set aside, doctors are still pivotal. It is doctors who are accessible or not, who are the primary purveyors of quality care (or lack of it), and who are paid with a huge percentage of the health care dollar. Doctors also determine how other big chunks of that dollar are spent on care through hospitalization, return appointments, referrals, testing, prescriptions, and use of advanced technology. Doctors even help determine who is entitled to disability payments. And doctors are the ultimate experts on virtually all clinical issues.

What group has the greatest responsibility to provide the most expert input and effective leadership for improving our nation's health care? To paraphrase a well-known expression from the Clinton campaign: "It's the doctors, stupid." What group has failed most with regard to improving care? Unfortunately, the answer is the same.

The Big Three: Cost, Quality, and Access

The cost of health care has been an issue at least as far back as the New Testament story of the woman cured of her hemorrhaging by Christ. This narrative relates how "she had endured much under many physicians, and had spent all that she had; and she was not better, but rather grew worse" (Mark 5:26, *The New Oxford Annotated Bible*). I found it interesting that during the preparation of "*Trust Me, I'm a Doctor*" an acquaintance related to me her own virtually identical personal story following a "D and C" procedure.

Debate will continue for years over the high cost of health care. But, high compared to what in our society? RVs? New cars? Entertainment? Vacations? What? The real issue isn't cost. It's what we expect to get for our dollar—and we'll surely get what we pay for in health care.

The situation is reminiscent of an old skit with Jack Benny playing his famous skinflint role. He was ordered by a hold-up man to surrender his money or lose his life. After a long pause, his response was, "I'm thinking it over!" Like the troubled Mr. Benny, we must look at our priorities. What is our thinking with regard to the price of health care?

None of this is to ignore an obvious and frequent target of critics of high cost: Physicians' income. I'm fully in favor of fair compensation for a doctor's efforts. However, much of the cost is related more to a controlled supply other than to long hours and demanding work. What if twice as many doctors made half as much money? To my thinking $60,000 to $100,000 per year still isn't bad compensation for vital and interesting work which most physicians profess to enjoy. I've heard of a heart surgeon making a half million dollars a year. What is "fair?"

Hand in glove with the question of cost are questions of access and of quality. Access ultimately comes down to having enough physicians and enough other professionals to do "doctor-like" work. There's a basic misconception that the current number of practicing physicians would be adequate if they weren't distributed so poorly and over-specialized. I propose to you that when there really are enough doctors, distribution will take care of itself as a result of the usual market forces. Starving doctors won't stay in affluent suburbs. They'll go where they can make a living and where they can practice their art. Those moving to rural areas might actually find a bonus in the form of an improvement in their lifestyles.

Having an increasing number of generalists won't greatly improve access—and it may even decrease it. Specialists are usually busy, hard-working professionals whose expertise often provides care more efficiently, with more safety, and with fewer false starts. Making primary care doctors the gatekeepers regulating access to more specialized services is no panacea. Patients may simply run the risk of spending more time with less qualified practitioners.

For those concerned that there's a coming "doctors glut" with too many physicians, ask yourself these questions: How long have you waited for recent appointments? How much time did the doctor spend with you?

In some ways, the question of quality is a much tougher one. What is quality? From whose perspective? At what cost? How can it be monitored, much less enforced? Quality is not some theoretical issue. It's as literally "life and death" as you can get. Health care can be dangerous—even lethal. There are obvious consequences of poor care. Many of these show up in mortality and morbidity figures. (Mortality refers to death; morbidity refers to problems short of death.)

Those who die are sometimes the lucky ones. The surviving victims of so-called "medical misadventures" are often condemned to diminished lives of disability and pain. These survivors of care enter only the morbidity figures.

I recall one of my pediatric teachers in medical school telling me that many a pediatrician has provided the final shove as yet "another little angel wings its ways to heaven." It's unfortunate that this quotation focused on pediatricians. Of all clinicians, those who help care for our children are among some of the most dedicated, available, and caring that I know. But, the general point of physician culpability which it illustrates is a valid one. We physicians have another name for these complications of treatments. We call them "iatrogenic," which is a nice euphemism for "we did it to the patient."

Success is usually more likely in cases of well-defined, acute, relatively simple problems that are nonetheless beyond the layman's ability to self-manage. Treatment for a pneumonia or for appendicitis might be good examples. And in some very complex and desperate situations—for example, needing an organ transplant or having severe multiple trauma from an auto accident—there are, indeed, medical miracles awaiting some of the patients.

It also helps to have only one illness at a time. A patient with several illnesses at one time can present a confusing picture even for a very competent physician or can make prescribing medications more complex and risky. Having an illness that requires only one drug (e.g., an infection which can be treated with a single antibiotic) is much better and safer than having a problem that requires multiple medications.

In a way, the system isn't even so bad. It's just so much *less good* than it could be. One reason for this is that the medical world hasn't taken the time or effort to adequately help patients work effectively with it. Perhaps doctors just don't know how to adequately work in a partnership with those they're charged with protecting. If they could learn to act in such a fashion, doctors might even start volunteering to go to high schools to teach a course which could be called "basic patientology."

Moving Forward

Throughout my career, I've laid a foundation for my own understanding. Much of this could be summed up in the following statements (some are my own thoughts and some are from my physician-teachers):

- The seat of the psyche is in the wallet.
- The seat of the psyche is in the heart.
- Doctors are no more or less human than anyone else.
- The truth is, no one knows what the truth is.
- Life may or may not be unfair, but it certainly is tough for *everyone*.
- Everything is connected to everything else.
- It's not a matter of *if* we die, but *when*.
- Health care will always be inherently expensive.
- Amid all the chaos, there must be—and is—some basic order in life.
- A physician's most important tool is a professional *relationship* with the patient.

These are not offered for their absolute correctness. This brief collection obviously contains both paradox and error (we sometimes *do* know the truth). It also contains some obvious truths which are included here simply for emphasis. In spite of their shortcomings, these statements contain the most "wisdom per word" applicable to health care as I've been able to gather in almost a lifetime within the world of medicine. They'll help you as you make this book part of your own personal medical journey.

As you embark, remember this additional word of caution: Doctors realize that no two medical situations are exactly the same, so they tailor their actions to each individual case. Readers wishing to use the material in this book are well advised to adopt a similar attitude. Don't use what doesn't fit your needs or isn't appropriate to your specific situation. And, use this information—when appropriate and possible—within your relationship with a trusted and competent physician.

. . .

Complex health care issues can quickly enter into our lives, virtually turning them upside down with little warning. An inadequate, uninformed, ill-planned, or unnecessarily passive response to these situations can yield devastating consequences. Don't let this happen to you.

"*Trust Me, I'm a Doctor*" can help. Part One of this book primarily explores an understanding of the subculture that is the Biz-Med Complex. Part Two provides practical information for taking action in appropriate clinical situations. Finally, Part Three helps look ahead to our personal health care and to opportunities for affecting our nation's care.

Perhaps a rallying cry will emerge for you from these pages: "Involve me! It's *my* health." If the medical community won't give you that involvement, *take it*. Your initiative may save your life.

CHAPTER 2

The First Step to Better Care: A *Framework* of Understanding

Pearl:
Health care can't be understood in isolation, but only as an inseparable part of the fabric of life in general.

The Painful Journey to Knowledge

Why? is question that can be asked of many health care situations. Why does one obstetrician call for a C-section while another recommends a normal delivery in a similar situation? Why does one side in a malpractice case involving a fatal medication reaction feel the doctor is to blame, while the other side sees only the unfortunate consequence of acceptable practice?

I maintain that an understanding of these situations is within the grasp of most non-medical people. But how?

People look at the innate complexity of scientific knowledge. They look at the seemingly incomprehensible delivery system through which that knowledge is translated into patient care. And they get an inkling of the struggle which would be involved in learning about health care. Not surprisingly, most don't know where to begin.

You could certainly try to bite right into either of the situations described above. Each episode could be the subject of analysis and speculation. You might gain some insights, but you would not end up with a comprehensive understanding of health care.

Alternatively, you might first try to deal with the building blocks which go into making up health care, including understanding ourselves and other people, the doctor-patient relationship, the underlying purpose of health care, the proper functioning of health care organizations such as hospitals and clinics, the information physicians use in reaching treatment decisions, a method patients can use to acquire their own clinical knowledge, and the process of empowerment.

It would also help to understand the meaning people give to their day-to-day lives, as well as the *perceptions* and *forces* which affect the behavior of patients and caregivers alike.

Obviously, gaining all of this understanding is a formidable task. None of us, neither patients nor physicians, can ever fully understand it all. However, there are approaches which enable most of us to grasp the essentials.

Gaining understanding is possible if the emphasis is primarily on understanding the broader "whys" of health care rather than on focusing on the numbers, the details, or even the specifics of treatment. Understanding the "whys" helps you to see a more comprehensive picture of the entire health care world. This newfound perspective can be applied in a number of ways: Patients can develop their own overall personal vision of what *they* want in their care. They can develop approaches to use in clinical situations ranging from the routine to the critical. They can be alert to the dangers and opportunities involved in diagnosis and treatment. And, they can intelligently advocate productive *changes* within the system.

This chapter will help you outline an approach for gaining the understanding you need to take action. Subsequent chapters will provide further details as well as practical applications.

The Value of a Wider Perspective

Health care involves a broad mix of such basic issues as life and death, suffering, responsibility and accountability, choices, empathy, appropriate and inappropriate treatment, economics, ethics, philosophy, law, and religion.

These factors are largely "people issues." But our care is delivered in a clinical setting. How do such non-clinical factors fit in? These so-called "soft" issues may have more influence on the outcome of your care than such hard scientific data as abnormal laboratory tests or positive physical findings.

For example, the quality and nature of obstetrical and gynecological care may be highly influenced by factors that are not strictly medical issues. What are the practitioner's views on family size, pre-marital sex, masturbation, sex selection, homosexuality, aggressive care for very premature infants, or abortion? How seriously are the symptoms of women taken? To what extent is the office practice efficiently organized to provide adequate time and resources needed for proper care? To what extent is it organized primarily for the benefit of the practitioner instead of the patient?

Non-clinical issues such as guilt and finances also affect such critical decisions as maintaining or removing life-support systems from a patient. How does the cardiac surgeon feel about doing bypass surgery on an otherwise healthy 80-year old patient? How will the *government* feel about paying for it? Will a physician suggest a C-section more out of fear of a lawsuit or because it's clinically indicated? Will this surgery be suggested because it pays more than a routine delivery?

The basic concept here is that issues of life and death, illness and suffering, extend far beyond the purely clinical sphere. How can you presume to deal successfully with health care without a broad understanding of the individuals who deliver and receive that care—and of the professional and lay organizations in which they encase themselves? How can health care professionals presume to help you without their own broad understanding? We need some sort of a foundation.

Defining a Psycho-Philosophy

Auto accidents, murder, heart attacks in young people, failed relationships—both inside and outside the world of health care, seemingly inexplicable things happen. If we don't utilize some consistent internal guidance system to help us make sense of them—a philosophy for our lives—we can easily run aground: perplexed, overwhelmed, confused, and inefficient.

Since physicians and others in the health care field deal so directly with life and all its drama, we'd hope that they, especially, would be aided by a clear personal philosophy. We'd expect them to have some well thought-out concepts with which to daily bridge the deep gaps between what's possible through modern medicine and what makes sense for a patient.

I hope you won't be too surprised or disappointed when I tell you that this frequently isn't the case. Doctors aren't any more or less likely than your accountant or plumber to be able to articulate a comprehensive, thoughtful philosophy. Who am I? Why am I here? Who are you? Why are you here? Don't expect all doctors to have thoughtful answers.

If you have been diagnosed as having a serious illness such as cancer, you're forced to deal with the realities of many issues which are not purely clinical: life and death, suffering, wisdom, love, hope, dependency, family, even money. For you, many of these concerns become very practical issues of personal survival and comfort. Your physician should be equipped to help you in your consideration of them. Even though he or she may not be a qualified financial advisor, a doctor should be attuned to the monetary impact that your illness will have on you and your family. Most importantly, your physician should understand his or her role in helping you to confront your own mortality.

Actually, there are at least three sets of psycho-philosophies (my term which recognized the frequent blurring between psychology and philosophy) involved in health care: (1) that of the caregivers, (2) that of the patients, and (3) that of the organizations that directly affect caregivers and patients alike—everything from the AMA to insurance companies, hospitals, patient self-help groups, and government. Physicians need to understand you. You need to understand them.

To ignore psycho-philosophy is to lose a great opportunity in understanding health care. With psycho-philosophy we can move from superficial knowledge on to useful insights. Without these insights, we miss knowing our "souls" and the "souls" of our caregivers and their organizations. Psycho-philosophy contains the raw material for our understanding of practical ways to better care. (Since organizations can't be truly philosophical, we're speaking somewhat metaphorically in their case.)

While this book isn't a philosophy or psychology text, it can't avoid these two disciplines. The remainder of this chapter will put forth a framework I use in my own thinking, teaching, and practice. Topics in subsequent chapters will draw upon this material. There's no suggestion that this approach fully answers the ultimate questions of life and death. But it *will* stimulate your thinking along those lines!

"Life's a Bitch..."

Let's start by discussing individuals, regardless of whether they are physicians, other members of the Biz-Med Complex, or just ordinary folk.

Almost everyone has heard the saying that "life's a bitch, and then you die." There is an element of truth here. But, I think a somewhat fuller picture is captured by this: "Life is full of pain and suffering and misery. Then—all too soon—it's over." Everyone has had his or her own share of difficulty in life—or they will if they live long enough. I don't mean to present a particularly pessimistic view. Life must actually be *pretty good* if it can "all too soon" be over. Life can be wondrously satisfying. But, it *is* a mixed bag.

Satisfaction in life is tied to achieving what each of us understands to be its meaning. For some, this is success defined by power and money ("Those who die with the most toys win.") This is an especially tempting route for physicians who often wield significant power and generate large incomes.

For some, the meaning of life is in the pursuit of excellence or beauty or art. For others, it is fulfilling their role as parent or spouse. Some will see it as serving God or humankind, or simply as doing one's best. For a number of people, this "meaning" is nothing more than our DNA telling us "copy me," thereby providing for the survival of our species. No doubt, there are many other possibilities as well.

In pursuing life's purpose as we each understand it, we all have the opportunity to express the basic goodness which I suspect is inherent in us all. Perhaps this would allow us to build a health care system based on selflessness, caring, and the acceptance of individual responsibility. Maybe.

Must We Suffer?

Despite the satisfaction people derive from life, "suffering" is inexorable a part of our lives. Suffering is a confusing but relevant concept, one that is central to an understanding of health care. If medicine is a business, it is less the business of money and power (or even of curing) and more properly the business of suffering and death.

The term suffering is not equivalent to pain, nor is suffering confined only to the patient. It is the mind's weighing of the burden of any physical or mental illness (or simply of our imperfect human condition). It can develop out of the fears, uncertainties, disappointments, worries, separations, anxieties, empathy, and feelings of vulnerability and loss of control which can result from ill-health or other misfortune.

Other people can suffer as much as or more than the patient. The family suffers as one of its members grapples with illness. Friends suffer as they see the distress of the patient and perhaps even anticipate their own losses as a result of the illness' effect on that relationship. In spite of the classic admonition, "Don't get emotionally involved," caregivers often suffer along with their patients.

Suffering and death are not necessarily our enemies; they are not always bad. Suffering is the natural fate of all of us. Death is not always to be feared or to be avoided at all costs.

It's important for you to understand that these comments are not made to encourage more suffering and deaths. Rather, I say this to provide some perspective on what will surely come to us all. As important as suffering and death are, they are *not* absolute enemies. My point is that there is not some simple equation of "good health care equals triumph over suffering and death."

Defining the Goals of Care

So, what *is* the purpose of health care?

Defining the goals of health care is a little like trying to define art or pornography: we may not be able to completely put it into words, but we usually know it when we see it.

"I want to feel better," is a fairly basic goal. Upon further scrutiny, we see that health care can be used in the prevention of illness or injury as well as for treatment. As I just implied, many people want it to prevent suffering and death. And, in our modern culture, there is ultimately the desire for health care to help develop a superbly functioning person who is physically and emotionally well. These goals, within limits, are all correct.

But, there *are* limits, and there are other goals. A significant limitation is that suffering and death cannot and should not always to be avoided. A significant goal—in fact, the most fundamental goal in health care—is to prevent *unnecessary* suffering and *premature* death. In addition, human beings are subject to frailties—ignorance, despair, fear, and isolation, as well as illness and injury.

Despite these limitations, the relationship between patient and caregiver can sustain both individuals in the face of human frailty. While our vulnerability is tremendous, so are our strengths. That we are simultaneously so very strong and so very weak is a paradox of health care.

Each of us can be described as having a core of physical and emotional vulnerabilities—such as debility or depression—which are poised to express themselves. We also have a strong protective shell around these which keep them contained. Although a vital role of all caregivers is to provide an antidote to these vulnerabilities, as well as to help strengthen the defensive shell, this is best achieved within the context of a healthy patient-doctor relationship.

A valid goal for all professionals *is* to help people feel better. But it's the epitome of the art of medicine to comfort the patient within the bonds of this special relationship. Through it, the vulnerabilities are diminished and the strengths are enhanced. While it's good to have someone fix your broken leg, it's even better to have someone by your side who understands how this accident affects you personally and emotionally, not just physically.

Most patients desire this kind of meaningful attachment to their healers. Unfortunately, patients don't always realize how their own understanding and power can enhance this vital relationship.

Physicians, on the other hand, know the value of their innate healing power, and this realization can help them be better healers. But, it can also contribute to a "god-like" comportment and arrogance.

Fear and ignorance both play roles as patients enter into a traditional covenant with their healers: "You take care of me—without too much inconvenience or involvement on my part—and

I will accord you a special status." For their part, these caregivers agree to function as tradition dictates: "Set me apart and I will use my powers on your behalf." Although the deal completely skews the balance of power and communication, people nevertheless feel more secure within this protective arrangement.

Even in its current flawed state, this relationship is at the very foundation of health care. But it is badly in need of renegotiation.

Rewiring the Relationship

The capabilities of doctor and patient for greater empathy is an extremely powerful influence for better care. They can bond with each other while striving together for the knowledge which will allow some control over human frailties. *Capability* can triumph over *vulnerability* in critical areas—everything from pneumonia to psychosis. It's no wonder that the patient-doctor relationship is so potent.

It's not enough for the doctor to merely "take care of" the patient. To totally fulfill this relationship, the patient must be empowered to actively participate. I'm reminded of an expression I often heard during my years in rural practice. Patients would sometimes talk of "doctoring with..." rather than of "going to the doctor." These people were on the right track.

A Three-Dimensional View

So far, I've presented a general view of how people participate in the patient-doctor relationship. But we can also take a more focused look to see why people—including those who deliver health care—behave the way they do. Ultimately, this knowledge will lead to better care.

Behavior is steered by significant influences which spring from three sources: reality, our perceptions, and forces which drive or motivate us. I call these the "Big 3 Influences."

The reality part of this triad is easy to understand: It is what actually happens in our lives, measured objectively.

Perceptions address the question: How do we see life and its problems, regardless of reality? Our perceptions, of course, can be as real to us as any reality. For example, you have as much joy in your life as you think you do, regardless of how joyful or joyless it may appear to an observer.

Forces are those factors which drive or motivate our lives and our organizations. Compassion and the financial "bottom line" are examples of such personal and organizational forces, respectively.

This chapter provides only the briefest general description of these perceptions and forces, plus some specific examples pertinent to health care. This is adequate, however, to follow the discussions in subsequent chapters. (For those who desire more detail, I've provided an "advanced course" in Appendix A.)

The simple message is that reality, along with the cumulative effects of certain perceptions and forces, has a tremendous impact upon us all. All three concepts can be combined to more fully understand what influences people in general—and, consequently, what influences them in the health care they provide or receive. Once we understand how these affect the delivery of our care, we have the basis for improving it.

Let's look at just a few examples of influences occurring in the medical world. I'll italicize specific perceptions or forces. First, consider perceptions. In their professional work, physicians see themselves in *control* (or wishing to be), not sharing the decision-making process with the patient. They combat their own scientific *ignorance* with a sometimes shaky belief system. They will work best with patients with whom there has been *bonding* within the relationship. But, doctors may put their own best interests first if they see their professional or financial *survival* threatened. For instance, a generalist might overstep his or her ability rather than lose a patient (and fee) to a specialist.

Patients will often feel inadequate to the task of meaningful participation in their care. They may see only their own *ignorance*, the apparent *chaos* of the system, and an enforced *passivity* in receiving care. Yet, their *control* of their own care may be critical to their very existence. In the depths of their illnesses, when *isolation* can be the most severe patients may need the *bonding* of the patient-doctor relationship all the more.

The significant effect of very strong personal forces influencing health care must also be understood. Both caregivers and patients must learn to recognize the role of *money*, *self-esteem*, and a sense of the *territorial*. For example, physicians with high self-esteem feel less threatened by actively participating patients. Patients with high self-esteem are less intimidated by physicians. Both physicians and patients who are less territorial will see options for care outside of the immediate formally structured environment, i.e. "alternative medicine."

The importance of money in health care can't be emphasized too strongly. Depending on financial resources, lives are saved and lost daily in the medical marketplace. Money influences prevention, diagnosis, treatment, and certainly attitude. When I was in psychiatry residency at Loyola in Chicago, a very wise teacher (Dr. Domeena Renshaw) brought this to my attention: The seat of the psyche is in the wallet. It was one of the most useful lessons I've ever had.

. . .

What about the very potent influences affecting organizations? I've been told that fear and greed are powerful forces in the business world's decision-making process. While there's some truth in this—even when applied to non-profit organizations—we can also develop a broader understanding of additional relevant forces which influence groups or organizations.

For example, *organizations need to be understood as a collection of individuals to be reckoned with one by one*, rather than as an amorphous corporate or bureaucratic mass. In health care, it's often more important to know particular nurses or doctors at an institution than to have knowledge of a hospital. (Similarly, most business people appreciate the importance of knowing a well-placed secretary rather than just being familiar with the firm.)

Organizations, like individuals, so value their existence that they will often *take uncharacteristic actions to survive*, including *changing their original mission*, thereby mutating into something far different. For example, hospitals are moving from providing inpatient care to offering more outpatient services. Likewise, the March of Dimes no longer focuses so much on polio, but on birth defects. Such adaptability isn't mentioned here to condemn these changes, but simply to help you understand more fully how health care organizations operate.

Also similar to people, hospitals want what is "theirs," and *often operate as if "more" and "bigger" are better*. Hospitals have traditionally worked on the premise that increasing the number of beds and buildings means that they are better hospitals. More recently, financial realities have taken precedence, requiring some of them to downsize.

. . .

In the remaining chapters of Part One, perceptions and the forces acting upon you, as well as on providers and health care organizations will be examined in order to understand many aspects of the industry, its patients, and its practitioners. In Part Two, this understanding will be put to practical use.

Before we move on, however, let me make this point: To accomplish much of what this book suggests will require understanding of yet another basic concept: change. Change is one of the most easily defined—and difficult to accomplish—aspects of our lives and our communities. It's also one of the most necessary.

If change were easy, life would be perfect. The poor could work to become rich, the fat would lose weight to become thinner, those unhappy in their careers would smoothly switch to a different field. Those who want to stop smoking or drinking would do so. Our nation would heal its racial strife. Of course, all of these changes are very, very difficult.

So, I know I am asking a lot when I suggest that patients start to become more actively involved in a health care system which they've traditionally approached with passivity. It's not easy to take responsibility for your own health when such responsibility has been routinely delegated to others for so long. And it certainly won't be easy to alter physicians' attitudes or to make more than cosmetic adjustments in our nation's health care spending patterns.

There are some ingredients, however, which can help provide a "climate for change": (1) a reasonably clear "vision" of the goal (which helps dispel fear of change), (2) adequate resources of time, money, people, skills, energy and technology, and (3) "fertile ground"—that is, a system which is flexible and strong, and in which the psychological cost won't be too great.

Some of these ingredients are already partially in place. There are practitioners and institutions who have a clear vision and who have pointed the way to the future. The same could be said of some patients who handle their health care quite well. And, we have the resources for change, provided we learn to effectively apply them.

What we may not have is sufficiently fertile ground to be able to cope with the necessary changes. We undoubtedly have the potential to do so. But history would cast some doubt upon the outcome.

Toward a Practical Application

In general, how is the leap made from understanding to better care? Such a move may involve a number of small hops. For example, knowing the weaknesses within a system alerts one to precautions that should be taken. Knowing the normal operation affords recognition when things go amiss. Knowing the potentials or possibilities avoids accepting inadequate efforts.

The ABCs of empowerment, introduced in Chapter 1, can work along with these hops. An "I-can-do-it" *attitude* encourages effort where appropriate. *Blueprints* such as the "Four Steps to Better Care" suggest practical approaches. And a *climate for change* provides fertile ground in which better care can occur.

People who *understand* the health care system need be less reliant on rigid, stereotypical responses. They can be creative and flexible as problems arise. This is important because no two situations are identical—and the way health care is delivered is changing rapidly.

As you continue, I offer this basic foundation for both patients and physicians: The most important factors to be understood in health care delivery are (1) people themselves and (2) their relationships with each other. Less important—but obviously still critical—is the clinical knowledge of physicians *and* patients alike.

CHAPTER 3

Understanding Doctors

Pearl:

No task—not even the most menial—should be beneath the dignity of the physician in caring for the sick.

Most physicians really do start out as idealists; many just don't end up that way. For these people, the journey from student to practitioner is simply too long and too arduous.

Under the best circumstances, their training is demanding, usually disruptive of normal life and personal development. It's often demeaning and disappointing, but it almost always has at least a financially successful conclusion. This education is provided in the context of a society only marginally idealistic itself. The result: The proverbial bright-eyed and bushy-tailed students frequently become the stereotypically arrogant and aloof physicians, insulated from the world they had hoped to serve.

The doctor-in-training undergoes a process more akin to manufacturing than learning. This trend is worsening as students are indoctrinated into the corporate ways of managed care. The product (a doctor) which is pressed out during the molding process yields little to later potentially corrective outside influences such as family and exposure to human frailty.

Medicine is not taught as a contemplative field. Medical faculty see health care more like a battlefield for an army of quick-moving, action-oriented practitioners. Doctors follow orders learned in medical school and residency. As the neophytes advance in training, they are equipped with more "realistic" and "practical" approaches to care. They get very good at making quick decisions and then acting upon them. Unfortunately, these choices are not always the correct ones.

The newly learned ways are not always in the patient's best interest. However, this may cease to be of concern to the doctor as idealistic images begin to fade. The attitude of "we patients and physicians *together*" of earlier student days can become an "us *versus* them" attitude.

Women students can suffer even more than male doctors-to-be in this transformation. You may not agree with me that women in our society are more nurturing and caring than are men. My experience dictates otherwise. Consequently, I feel that a woman's journey is even more difficult and more painful in a profession still dominated by male values.

(For simplicity, physicians will often be referred to as "he" and "his" or "him." This convention should not be construed as denying the acknowledged—and sometimes even superior—abilities of women physicians.)

For doctors of either sex, how does this negative transition occur? There's no organized malevolent conspiracy. Instead, there is a subtle interaction of several factors: the physician's emerging psychology, the pressures of an inefficient educational system and of an equally inefficient production-oriented professional world, and the trends and deterioration of the larger society of which the medical world is a part.

Many practitioners accept the resulting trade-off. They wish to be special, to be apart from the rest of the world. I think that this attitude is captured in one of my favorite doctor jokes, given here in abbreviated form: A well-known, but arrogant, physician died during busy office hours. He became angered over both his inconvenient demise and subsequent long wait in line for celestial processing. After complaining to St. Peter at the Pearly Gates, he was told that even doctors must wait their turn to get into heaven. The physician acquiesced until he saw a distinguished-looking gentleman with a stethoscope and white coat walk through the portal without any delay. When he again protested, St. Peter assured him, "That was just God. He likes to pretend he's a doctor."

Almost no one else receives the combination of intellectual privilege, opportunity to serve, and even the chance for wisdom which is given to physicians. This is not to deny that knowledge or wonder awaits the student physicist, astronomer, English teacher, secretary, artist, or actor. But a special blessing is in store for those who study how life unfolds and then assist in its progress. They can marvel first-hand at a most wonderful and complex creature: the human being. They have society's permission—indeed, mandate—to peer into each and every crevice and cavity of the mind and body. They are anointed by the larger society which they are to serve. Indeed, physicians and society enter into an almost religious, but largely unspoken, covenant.

. . .

There are many circumstances which put a person on the road to being a physician. At one extreme are those who are almost pre-ordained by virtue of membership in a medical family; at the other end are reasonably bright people who must choose to "be something." Between the extremes are any number of circumstances. But for all these people, there is usually an underlying mindset of service. A desire to help people is more than just a cliché, for many it's a very real goal.

But before the final decision is made, all manner of additional factors get stirred into the pot, including issues of prestige, control, and cash.

The Training Years

The road to an M.D. degree is a bumpy one. Beginning in college with pre-medical courses, students start on the path to isolation and narrowness. Much of an individual's normal adult development and maturity will have to be postponed until his late 20s or even 30s.

Many doctors may never know what it's like to hold a "real" job. After medical school and residency training, they essentially start at the top in terms of position and prestige—often with huge incomes.

Doctors have great job security; once in practice, they rarely need worry about being fired or otherwise unemployed. They have superiors to report to only in a very limited fashion (for example, to the chairman of their department if something goes very wrong clinically or to a licensing board if they act with gross inappropriateness). A great deal of marginal behavior may be accepted by their colleagues, patients, and hospitals.

Likewise, physicians' non-professional contact with real people and the real world is often extremely limited. You usually won't find doctors riding the buses, in trouble with creditors, brown-bagging in the cafeteria, or socializing with factory workers or salespeople.

While still in college, the world of the pre-med student is more focused on laboratories, books, classrooms, study, securing enough financing to finish their education, and competing to stay on top so as to get that all-important acceptance letter into medical school. While other students socialize, work, and experience the world around them, typical pre-med students will dissect, memorize, and go to never-ending classes and labs. Great literature takes a back seat to the dissection of cats.

Pre-med students work like little demons. They desperately want to be physicians. They want it to the extent that without an M.D. in their future, they hardly see any future at all. There may well be more than just a little psychopathology in this attitude. If they fail to get into a U.S. medical school, they'll often head to Mexico, the Caribbean, or wherever they can accomplish their goal. The hardships endured even in the U.S. can be tremendous. After all this effort, its not surprising that doctors find it difficult to be critical of the profession.

. . .

What does it take to become a physician?

Medical schools maintain what they see as high standards for admissions. This is in spite of the fact that some students aren't even interviewed prior to acceptance. The primary standard is grades and admission exam results.

Ironically enough, obtaining top grades really shouldn't be that significant. This may come as a surprise to you, but about 90 percent of medical school involves such relatively simple activities as memorization, dissection of a cadaver (which is more labor-intensive than challenging), and repetitive types of work on hospital wards. Students do standard patient examinations, put in I.V.'s, make daily notes on the patients' charts, collect specimens—with the more menial tasks often referred to as "scut work."

A student's knowledge base can be a hit-and-miss affair. Physicians can enter practice having learned little about much. For instance, they can be almost totally ignorant of problems associated with "post-polio" or of the value of psychotherapy. While they may see a lot of death, they are taught very little about dying. Only a small percentage of students' work may actually require serious understanding and abstract thinking. Occasionally, they may be faced with some truly intellectual challenges. These include the times of ethical considerations, treatment dilemmas, philosophical concerns, and creativity.

What medicine should require for admission to its ranks are candidates who understand the world about them and who have a proven track record of successful interaction with others. An ideal candidate would be a reasonably bright person who has first spent some years in the trades, business world, nursing profession, or childrearing.

I don't think medical studies necessarily require much more than a slightly higher than normal I.Q.—along with the time and energy to master the material and do the work. Of course, students also need the money which makes it all possible. They often build up huge debts during their pre-practice years. This worries them. Actually, they shouldn't be so concerned. Just about any investor would be ecstatic to receive the kind of financial return most students can expect.

Medical schools need to place less of an emphasis on technical and scientific issues, and more on people, caring, and character issues. Medicine is still an art, but doctors have become technicians. I'm not saying that they don't need a reasonable level of smarts—they do. But, on the balance, given an acceptable level of intelligence in all candidates, I'd pick the ones who were "people-oriented." Then I'd see to it that they were taught the clinical knowledge and skills they need.

In the "old days," prospective students generally had to have high I.Q.s, the presence of male genitalia, the ability to conform to a rigid system, and access to money. The more naive and inexperienced they were in dealing with life, the better. We're seeing some positive changes currently. For instance, the percentage of women and minority students has markedly increased. Even older students are being accepted. Now, if this "new breed" can only keep its perspective...

. . .

What is the nitty-gritty of daily medical school life like? While there is some variation from school to school, mostly it's a matter of fitting into the system—or leaving it.

The first two years of medical school are called pre-clinical years. They are largely academic, consisting of classroom and laboratory work in areas such as anatomy and physiology. The next two years, called the clinical years, are divided into periods of practical experience or clerkships. During this latter time, the student doctor will primarily work in hospital units such as surgery, OB, pediatrics, and so on. Bookish, more introspective students, can do well the first two years. But they seem to turn the lead over to the more aggressive and "action-oriented" students in the last two years on the wards. This is because students generally are taught that to do *something* is the ideal; to be a physician, one must "phys-ish" (pronounced "fiz-ish"). This generally means to take action. Yet, that's not always in the patient's best interest. One of the more difficult concepts to teach students is captured in the saying, "don't just do something, stand there."

Clerkship experiences vary widely for students. They often serve under the direction of residents. Residents, in turn, are already M.D.s, but are receiving additional training, called "residencies," in obstetrics, pediatrics or other specialties. So the medical students become students of other students (the residents).

When on the wards, students may look, act, and dress like doctors. Some will even refer to themselves as "Doctor", but don't let yourself be fooled. Look at that name tag very carefully. Does it specifically say "M.D." or "D.O.?" (D.O. means Doctor of Osteopathy. These days, medical students and osteopathic students essentially receive equally rigorous training.)

Depending upon the circumstances and settings, the amount of clinical "practice" which students get differs markedly. At public facilities such as state or county hospitals, they generally are given (by default, due to inadequate staffing) more actual responsibility, including decision-making. They also do more things directly to the patient, such as starting I.V.s, putting in bladder catheters, and even doing spinal taps. It's in these public sector settings that a "see one, do one, teach one" approach to training reaches its greatest expression. If you're the patient being "done to," it's not necessarily an ideal situation.

In private facilities, students may have more of a hands-off approach. Here, private attending physicians are caring for private paying patients. These patients (or more likely, their insurers) are paying big bucks for treatment. They are more inclined to expect care from the real doctors. And the real doctors feel more of a vested interest in private patients in order to maintain their loyalty and to avoid malpractice suits.

It's during the clerkship experience that students start learning all is not well within the system. They observe deceptive practices and out-and-out cheating. They see patient examination reports appearing on the charts for exams they know weren't performed. They see patients operated upon with assembly-line precision, and sometimes with about as much humanity. And they hear talk of dishonest billing practices.

In spite of all the problems, there are many positive aspects of the clerkship experiences. Students are exposed to massive numbers of patients. And it is true that "we learn from our patients." A real patient suffering a real heart attack is a much more educational than a textbook discussion about heart attacks.

The students pick up skills such as suturing, delivering babies, and holding retractors at surgery. They learn to be comfortable in situations and conversations far from normal social interaction ("How many tampons do you use per day, Ms. Smith?") and how to perform under great pressure. The students learn to exist in a world of body parts, feces, urine, pus, human tissue, and blood. They start fearing for their lives as they work with AIDS patients. They learn the necessity of being able to tolerate the presence of people in very severe pain. That is, they become acculturated into the medical environment—hopefully into a "culture of healing."

Equally significant is what students don't learn. Medical education lacks much of the careful structuring and systematic checks of knowledge which I see in aviation training. Medical students may or may not be taught a specific clinical topic; if taught, they may or may not be tested on it.

Even more important than the content of their training is the way in which the students are psychologically incorporated into the system. If medicine were a cult, we would probably call this training "brainwashing." Tired and confused, the students are offered camaraderie and acceptance in exchange for buying into the system. They learn that hard work and long hours as laborers in the vineyard bring praise and good grades. It's best to not make waves. If they'll line up with their teachers against the lawyers, administrators, bureaucrats, and non-M.D. professionals such as psychologists and even nurses, they'll do well. Slowly and insidiously, the student's focus shifts from the patient's needs to personal needs for rest and reward; for some free time and recognition; for power and acceptance. Positive role models are often conspicuous by their absence.

If students can accomplish three tasks, they're allowed to graduate. These obstacles are (1) pleasing the faculty, (2) passing exams, and (3) learning to take care of patients. The three aren't necessarily closely related.

. . .

After medical school graduation, acculturation continues in specialty training programs known as residencies and fellowships. Five or six additional years of work aren't unusual. Residents experience more long hours, more memorizing, more fatigue, more isolation, and frequent "call." Call means working extra hours to be available for emergencies and even routine work, such as ordering sleeping pills for restless patients or pronouncing patients dead. It can result in the resident working 36 hours or more straight—

sometimes doing the equivalent of a week's work without stopping. I remember an incident during my residency in psychiatry when I fell asleep during a therapy session after a night on call. The patient had to awaken me.

There's a saying that the only really bad thing about being on call every other night is that you still miss half of the good cases. The faculty benefits tremendously from having their residents work such long hours; residents are understandably less enthusiastic. But this is part of their "initiation" (although today it is now getting some of the scrutiny given to the "hazing" that occurs in other fraternities).

The Practice Years

Finally, the big moment comes. The residency period is over. Instead of being the performer of "scut," the doctor is now sought after by clinics, hospitals, and even entire communities. An overnight celebrity, he is wined and dined until he signs.

For his services, big bucks await him. Starting salaries between $100,000 and $200,000 aren't unusual. (And, the institutions with which he affiliates benefit even more, from charges for room occupancy, operating room use, laboratory tests, various therapies, and many other services and products.)

By the time his financial courting begins, the physician is often beaten and bruised. He brings into the negotiations an isolation from the rest of the world, insecurity in what he has been taught, uncertainty as to his medical potency, a "circle the wagons" mentality, and a willingness to exchange dollars for independence. Occasionally, even ethics are sold out at the bargaining table. The doctor can become the front man for corporations marketing their medical services. In managed care settings, the physician will have to decide in whose best interest clinical decisions will be made—and the patient won't always come first.

The mind, being both a wonderful and a terrible thing, must deal with this transformation in progress. When the truth is too painful, the mind can simply refuse to see it, refuse to think about it. And the mind can be far from benevolent. As it works to adapt to difficult situations, for instance being required to see too many patients in too little time, day after day, it charges for its services. The cost of this mental transformation can be a new approach toward patients: the doctor often moves from compassion, spirituality, and caring, to arrogance, worldliness, coldness, and aloofness. Like his patients, he too may even start to feel powerless. Many physicians could use a good dose of empowerment themselves in order to properly exercise their own appropriate responsibility and authority.

. . .

Eventually, the doctor decides where to locate his practice. This is done on the basis of many factors. Anticipated income, impressions of one's potential colleagues and practice, and physical attributes of an area (mountains, seashore, and so on) are certainly some of the most commonly considered ones. Additional issues are group vs. solo practice, rural vs. urban life, public vs. private sector. These issues and many others all figure into the final equation.

All too often the needs of the family (especially the spouse) are left in the dust of the decision-making process. From virtually everyone's perspective, the belief seems to be that if the doctor in the family is happy, *all* will be happy. This attitude can set the stage for future family tragedy.

. . .

After the move, the doctor starts to settle comfortably into his day-to-day schedule. A benefit of a medical life is that there is a reassurance brought on by a familiarity which flows throughout the doctor's environment. Despite obvious superficial differences, a hospital is a hospital, a medical office and its staff are still a medical office and its staff. Even an operating room at Ivory Tower Medical

Center may not look significantly different from an operating room in Small Town, U.S.A.

This sameness is part of the reason that physicians are often inadequately introduced to the specific functioning of their new environments. It's not unusual for doctors reporting for work their first day to simply be pointed toward the patients without receiving adequate indoctrination. This would rarely happen to pilots, executives, or nurses.

Typical days for the young physician start early and end late. The routine often begins with one of the most sacred of a series of daily medical rituals: making rounds. This is when the doctor visits hospitalized patients (usually referred to possessively as "my patients"). Other major rituals include doing surgery (for those trained in the appropriate specialties), seeing patients at the office, and being on-call.

Rounds present one of the greatest opportunities both for healing and for showmanship—especially if students or residents are in tow. The patient's physician (called "the attending" in teaching institutions) can simultaneously teach and humiliate the trainees. Bits of precious clinical information are sometimes called "pearls." But the attending physician often behaves as if he is casting these to the swine. (I hope it's with a more positive attitude that I'm including my own "pearls" in this book.)

Rounds may begin at the nurses' station with a report from a nurse. This is a summary for the doctor of the patient's problems and progress since the previous report. The value of this activity can be tremendous—with the opportunity for exchanging life-saving information. Usually it lives up to this expectation, but sometimes degenerates into a useless ritual (a perfunctorily tossed out "no change") or into a basically social encounter between doctor and nurse.

Following report, it's time for the usually brief—but expensive—visit with each patient. Many smart physicians use this time to literally perform a laying on of hands, being certain to touch each individual. This might be done by means of taking the pulse, palpating (medical-ese for feeling) the belly, or simply a pat on the shoulder (sometimes facetiously known as "upper deltoid therapy").

Some doctors are very good about interacting with patients. Others are like sleeping cats who must be prodded into action to respond to the patient's requests and needs. These latter physicians would often rather "treat the chart"—that is, they proceed more on the basis of information in the record (nurses' notes, test reports, and so on) than by talking with and examining the patient.

The level of severity of illness in patients seen on rounds has escalated over the years. Patients perceived as less ill now often aren't even allowed admission to the hospital. Those who do qualify for admission generally stay for shorter periods. Regardless of need, the doctor's time is often very limited for answering questions or offering reassurance.

The terminally ill have the roughest time maintaining the doctor's attention. This may be because of the doctor's perceived sense of his own failure with them or what might be seen as the clinical futility of working with them. Whatever the reason, time is often particularly short with this group.

After the completion of rounds, the doctor may be on to surgery. If the medical world has a *sanctum sanctorum*, it is the O.R. (operating room). Here, only the high priests and acolytes enter. The surgeon's hands are purified by a ritual-like washing and scrubbing prior to admission. He is then "gloved" and ceremoniously gowned in his vestment prior to cutting. The passwords for admission to the O.R. are "Doctor" or "Nurse." Patients are obviously also admitted, but often only once they are pre-medicated and groggy. Even then, they may be promptly put right "to sleep."

The O.R. is the site of one of the most efficient efforts in the medical world. Here, the lines of authority are about as clear as one can get, and everyone has a job to do. Generally, the surgical team works together quite smoothly. An occasional surgeon's tantrum may be the only disruptive activity marring the procedure. Sometimes either popular music from the radio or sexist banter from the operating team belies the seriousness of the situation as the incision is made. But the mood is generally appropriately professional. The work can be long, tedious, and even physically demanding.

Surgeons are often compared to the captain of a ship. They have absolute authority in the operating room. None dare defy their every request, their every decision. The major difference, of course, is that these captains won't go down if the ship does.

After surgery is finished, the physician may visit the medical records room. This chore is generally seen as a necessary evil. Medical records is a place to be avoided. The doctor sees his time there as unproductive: curing no one, charging no one. Still, regulations demand his presence. Sometimes the records staff will try to lure him in with promises of coffee and snacks.

In the records room, signatures are placed on vital documents with often nary a glance as to content. These important papers are primarily typed reports of operations, history and physical examinations, or summaries of patients' hospital stays. Or they may be orders given verbally days or weeks earlier to a nurse, but now awaiting the confirming imprimatur of the doctor.

Next, he may visit the Radiology Department to look at patients' X-rays; go on to the Emergency Room to see a patient who needs more immediate attention or specialized equipment than an office visit would provide; or go to the doctors' lounge. While not quite as holy as the O.R., the lounge is much more exclusive. Patients are not allowed in at all and non-M.D. staff is only briefly tolerated as they perform necessary tasks. Here, amidst coffee, sweet rolls, and mail, an important bond of collegiality is developed and expressed between physicians. Here—for a few comfortable minutes—fears are aired, commiseration provided, and social plans are made. It's really a support group. Then, it's on to the office.

. . .

The office is surely the feudal manor of the doctor, and he is its lord. Activities here are focused much less on direct patient care than might be imagined. This is because the office is also a center for paperwork, personal business decisions, professional study, more collegiality with peers, banter with the nurses, and the doctor's phone contact with his family—sometimes as a substitute for personal involvement with them.

It's also a center for the doctor to get his dose of ego massage and a modicum of social life. In short, it is just about like any other feudal manor. Unfortunately, it frequently shields the doctor further from the real world in which his patients live rather than adding to his understanding of peoples' day-to-day struggle.

To reign safely and efficiently in this manor, the doctor must be protected. His guards are his staff: receptionist, nurse, secretary, and others. They can be as impenetrable as the closed ranks of a battle line. For patients to breech the line, they may need luck, acceptability in the eyes of the staff, assertiveness, an adequate level of pain or suffering to merit attention, financial resources, the proper referral from another doctor, or knowledge of the right symptom buzz-words, such as "seizure," "severe abdominal pain," "suicidal thoughts," "bloody urine," and so on. Words like "tired," "back pain," "flu," or "another headache" may not pass muster—at least, not if the patient wishes to be seen promptly.

The office staff is usually exclusively female. Regardless of their age or function, they are generally referred to as "the girls." Strangely, this is frequently not instituted by the doctor, but rather by the staff members themselves.

In the office, the doctor rarely has any downtime, although not all efforts are patient-related. If any waiting is to be done, it will be done by the patients. Although both he and his staff are well aware of the predictable non-patient activities mentioned above, the appointment book will probably not take these into account. It may be tightly filled from start to finish.

The modus operandi of the office is rarely explicitly articulated, but is nevertheless clear to patient and staff alike. It is this: the doctor's time is precious. Within the office, the world will revolve around his schedule. He shall not be delayed or inconvenienced by anyone—especially patients. (An exception to this is pharmaceutical company representatives.)

Tightness of scheduling with little time allowed for emergencies, has at least two consequences. First, the resulting full waiting room clearly shows (perhaps unintentionally) just how important the doctor must be. Secondly, the doctor will always have a steady stream of business. He won't have to stand around even for a few minutes.

. . .

Finally, the doctor and the patient meet. The physician is in his white coat. The patient—often in some stage of undress—is usually addressed as just plain "Bill" or "Susie," depending on who is involved in the conversation: Rarely will you hear a "Mr.," "Ms.," "Miss," or "Mrs." The patient is essentially physically and psychologically naked. In this very unequal encounter, the doctor is, of course, known as "Doctor" (which I think is proper, but it is simply unreciprocated).

Visits can be stressful for the doctor as well as patient. Every patient is a potential adversary—a malpractice suit just waiting to happen. Subsequent to the visit, patients may experience any number of unpreventable complications from their illness or its treatments—or other problems which are totally unrelated to care. But, similar to a spouse in a murder case, the physician will often be the prime suspect in the minds of the patients or families until proven innocent.

A patient and doctor earnestly working together to relieve that patient's suffering can be an experience of joy and satisfaction for both parties. It's only proper to point out that some physicians facilitate this *very well*. The trick for patients is to find them.

During the office visit, the doctor will largely rely on all the facts and figures, dosages and procedures, he memorized in his training days. Information is rarely looked up. This is a matter of expediency, necessity, vanity, and denial all rolled into one. (The details of the very unique clinical encounter which is the office visit—and how a patient can get the most out of it—will be discussed in Chapter Ten, "The Doctor's Appointment.")

Throughout the day, phone messages from patients are delivered to the doctor. His response is often a prescription called in to a pharmacy or instructions for the patient to appear in the office at a time convenient to the doctor.

Occasionally a drug "detail man" (these days, this is often a woman) will appear unannounced and will be seen. Detail men or "reps" are the pharmaceutical version of the traveling salesman. He'll tell the doctor of the latest medication—"miracle" or not—brought forth by his company, but doesn't actually sell anything to him.

It's been an unwritten tradition that the detail man can be seen without an appointment. He may leave scientific literature, samples, and pens with advertising, as his price for admission—and as a reminder of which brand to prescribe. These sometimes abused folks are usually pleasant, knowledgeable, and patient people. While they'll often get seen without an appointment, they still spend a great deal of time in the waiting room.

. . .

The office day can typically end anytime between 5 p.m. and 7 p.m. The irregularity of its conclusion is often the rule rather than the exception. Regardless, "the girls" are expected to stay until the end.

Office hours may be over, but being on-call can continue. Departure from the office can simply mean a return to the hospital. The doctor can be on call for a number of reasons: to cover (i.e., be available for) his own practice, to alternate coverage with colleagues, to provide coverage to the emergency room of the hospital where he is on staff, or to back-up residents who may actually see the patient and do the work.

Call can last for a day, a week, or be just about always and forever—for instance, if the doctor is the only representative of his specialty in town (perhaps he is the lone neurosurgeon). Doctors are not typically paid for being available on-call, only for the services they render during that time. Some find that taking call is a blessing in building up a practice; others find it a curse—an intrusion on their already limited time.

If a patient is cared for by a doctor at the end of a long stint on-call, or by one who is on-call only because he must be, that patient should be prepared for the strong possibility of less than optimum care—or a sour attitude. (This is part of the reason patients are better off being seen by their own physician on a non-emergency basis if it is feasible.) Depending on circumstances, a doctor will often try to get out of taking care of an on-call patient. If he can't shift the responsibility to some other physician on the staff ("sounds like the cardiologist should see him"), he might try to "dump" him on some other facility. Doctors have many reasons—some quite valid—for instituting transfers (sometimes called "turfing"). For example, a burn unit at another hospital might offer advantages to a seriously burned patient.

Sandwiched amongst all these duties are any number of other activities. The physician is often volunteer to school sports teams, educator to the community, and server on both professional and civic committees. Many physicians spend long hours in independent study at home or travel to courses for their own continued professional growth. Trying to keep up is almost impossible for family doctors who must cover huge areas of knowledge. Specialists usually have a little easier time of it, but still must know the proverbial "more and more about less and less."

. . .

Eventually, the doctor arrives at home. For those physicians who have survived the psychological arrows of training and practice life, the home provides a welcome refuge. The care and concern which physicians dispensed during the day can be replenished by a caring family environment. The skewed world of the suffering and the dying, of experiences far outside the routine of most people's daily lives, can now be realigned by more normal human endeavors and encounters.

But if the doctor (or his family) has sustained more significant psychological damage during the process of his training and practice, the home can be an uncomfortable and threatening environment. To compensate for this, professional life often replaces home and family in the psychology of these physicians. They can't tolerate being perceived by family as the ordinary mortals they are. They feel that their supremacy shouldn't end at the threshold. Years of neglect of the family's emotional needs extract a horrible price in terms of divorce, problem children, and the doctor's unhappiness with life in general.

Often, medical marriages were founded on shaky premises. For instance, a bride- or groom-to-be may see a doctor (or future doctor) as especially desirable and dependable. She or he may be willing to overlook current flaws or even the potential for serious future problems that can befall medical families.

Many women have put their physician-husbands through school, only to see them married years later to someone who is younger and perceived as more attractive. There is even a facetious saying among physicians which recognizes this sad reality: "A doctor's first wife doesn't count." (I don't have enough information yet to comment about a doctor's first *husband.*)

By the time of the divorce, the spouse has often sacrificed much in the name of the doctor's career. Moves to various parts of the country are often dictated by the career, taking the spouse away from friends, family, preferred environment, and educational or personal career opportunities.

The saddest aspect of this family turmoil is the loss of potential. Far too few physicians are able to convert knowledge, intelligence, dedication, and financial advantages into personal and family satisfaction. Nor are they able to draw adequate beneficial replenishment from a nurturing family. How sad it all is—years of effort by the entire family are followed by personal disaster for all involved: abuse, unhappiness, divorce, dislocated families, and more. These days, parents would have to seriously ask themselves, "Would you want your daughter or son to marry a doctor?" Maybe not.

. . .

So, what is the basic psychology of the doctor? The simple answer is that doctors value what most other people do. The doctor wants to have meaning in his life, to be loved, to strive for excellence, to live long and happily (and these days, you can usually add wealth to that wish list). Unfortunately, these are all seen from the skewed perspective of a medical life.

Like other caregivers, physicians enter into a collective and unconscious pact with society. Doctors want the power and prestige of their elite profession, laying claim with some validity to a task that they propose only their select members can perform. Society wants care which will be virtually perfect, yet not be too significant a drain on its financial resources or personal energy. People want protection from their vulnerabilities. Even if our society realizes all this isn't possible to the desired degree, it will settle for a covenant that doctors will maintain the fantasy.

Society fulfills its part of the bargain by setting physicians apart with only minimal hassle—a little regulation, an occasional malpractice suit, a few spurts of bad press. Physicians promise what they can't deliver—an aura of availability, essentially limitless expertise, and consistent curing. The deal is struck. The doctors are satisfied and society gets a poor facsimile of the care it bargained for—or perhaps, deserves.

The typical scenario might go as follows: See a doctor for ten minutes with a complex problem, get reassurance and a prescription, and don't complain too much. "Mrs. Smith, you're just a little depressed. Cheer up. This Prozac should help." Both sides see their needs met. But the price is ultimately paid in terms of our current chaotic system and—at times—personal catastrophe.

In spite of their participation in this somewhat unholy alliance, physicians generally shouldn't be perceived as much better or worse than most other people. A major difference between the doctor and other people is that the doctor has often made particular decisions and had specific exposures throughout his life which have eventually led him into the medical world. Once he becomes a part of that world, he has greater opportunity than most people to do a job upon which society places a very high value: To work caringly in the service of relieving suffering and preventing premature death. Only to the extent that he fulfills this goal is any greater personal respect due the physician.

Another significant difference is that the focused, demanding education and training of physicians propels them along a track which largely obscures the world beyond themselves. They become separated from much of the reality of the lives of those they serve. As a consequence, doctor and patient emotionally move further and further apart. Both lose.

Additionally, doctors find that clinical cases are not so cut-and-dry in the real world as in the classroom and library. Patients apparently don't read the textbooks before developing their symptoms. Treatments don't work as effectively as promised. The better physicians will then realign their thinking to take into account what they don't know, as well as what they do know. Lesser physicians might react with arrogance and a "know-it-all" attitude. Regardless, practitioners find that patients get dissatisfied, families get angry, and lawyers help sue.

Doctors often exist in an exclusive ghetto of their own choosing with their own technically competent, well-to-do, but embattled peers. They see themselves as attacked by lawyers, bureaucrats, administrators, and even patients. They can slip into an isolated existence, largely devoid of philosophical concerns, variety, humility, or real financial problems. It is an existence which promotes the question, "Where's mine?" What is "mine" is often large homes, boats, expensive club memberships (which serve to further isolate), fancy cars, and even aircraft. It all might be described as "Lifestyles of the Rich and Medical."

While the doctor is usually perceived of as being independent in nature, the opposite is often true. He often seeks out a paid position, partnership in an established practice, corporate duties, or work with governmental agencies. The desire for an independent lifestyle gives way to the security of a large income and/or the power and prestige of affiliation with prominent organizations.

But to whom the gods give much, they extract a terrible toll. Physicians are not immune to the same psychological disruptions which can affect other people: depression, anxiety, excessive drinking, inappropriate sexual activity, feelings of extreme isolation, and all the rest. The difference is that these problems can become a hazard for their patients as well as for themselves. Impaired practitioners can become dangerous: Their skills are diminished, their knowledge outdated, and they take unnecessary risks. Perhaps worst of all they lose the energy and commitment necessary for a physician's contribution to a healing patient-doctor relationship.

. . .

Before leaving a chapter devoted to "Understanding Doctors," it would be appropriate to extend that understanding to physicians' legitimate professional role. If it appears that I've been rough on my medical colleagues, this discussion may explain why.

I hold the concept of "physician" in the highest regard. The fulfillment of all the potential that word conveys borders on the noble. Just imagine: In the time of your greatest need, at the time you are most vulnerable, there is someone to stand honorably with you in your suffering. There is someone to comfort, to relieve, to cure if possible. There is someone who will not take unfair advantage and who will protect confidentiality. There is someone who understands what is happening to you.

Still, the nobility of the physician is largely within the person, not the job description. A conscientious garbage collector who honorably performs a necessary service for society can be far more noble than an uncaring physician.

The physician's special responsibility can be seen in two general areas. First is to be the pre-eminent authority on the practice of medicine. Within this context, he is to forge a relationship which is nurturing, healing, empathetic, and empowering of the patient—professional in all ways. Second is to provide leadership to the patient, to students learning the art, and to society in demonstrating a respect for human life and in showing a path to the caring delivery of services to all citizens.

So, what is the bottom line in regard to physicians? On the one hand, it's that they must be held to an extremely high standard which promotes the finest in care. On the other hand, they are as human—and fallible—as anyone else. If a single word summed up physicians' best quality, it would be "caregiver," while "arrogant" captures the worst.

I'm not suggesting that physicians always live up to the positive expectations expressed in this section. We are prone to the same misperceptions and negative forces as other people—perhaps even more so. Still, it is worth striving toward the nobler goals. The first step toward better understanding between doctor and patient may be found within the admonition, "Physician, heal thyself."

. . .

Now, you've had a quick glimpse at "what makes the doctor run." You understand a little more of his practice and his life. That information is convertible into the coin of more productive interactions between patient and physician. Part Two of this book ("Getting Better Care") will provide many examples of application for obtaining that care. You'll see what a powerful tool you have in your understanding of what lies behind your care—especially the care by your physician.

CHAPTER 4

Understanding Hospitals

Pearl:

Hospitals should be vessels for the safe journey of lives in the balance, not simply monuments to modern science.

Hospitals are mysterious places. They represent a virtual subculture of our society, possessing their own language, customs and costumes, knowledge base, architecture, rituals, hierarchy, rules and taboos, commerce, and even outlying colonies. Like any culture, they can be capable of great good, or terrible harm.

Limited access and electronic equipment beyond comprehension help establish the alien atmosphere of these medical enclaves. Patients enter these technological wonderlands as veritable foreigners, often frightened and confused. Such intimidating institutions need to be understood, humanized, and rededicated to their critical mission: the best interest of a suffering human being in medical need.

What marvelous places hospitals can be! Marvelous, that is, if they are prepared to receive and participate with patients in the relief of their suffering. Many hospitals would claim that they are already doing this in caring and compassionate ways; patients and their families don't always agree.

Even though these institutions have been developed by society to be caring, within them patients often feel alone, as if they were burdens. This feeling can frequently be confirmed through over-heard staff conversations in elevators and cafeterias, in which patients are spoken of as if they were troublesome objects, not as people who need help.

To reap maximum benefits from hospitals in today's health care climate, you need to first understand their operation and their psychology. To start, here are four important general concepts to keep in mind when thinking of hospitals:

1. Hospitals, like most aspects of health care, largely have become businesses.

2. Their business is based on our suffering and dying.

3. They're often not very efficient at running their business—and, too frequently don't provide a service of adequate quality.

4. Unless patients, physicians, and hospitals work together, there's little chance of successfully developing a proper healing environment.

It's also important to differentiate between illness and suffering. Consider this: A man gets up on the morning of a scheduled routine medical exam. He has no known medical problem and is feeling happy and healthy. There certainly isn't any suffering occurring. A cancer is found during that day's examination. Nothing at all has changed except the patient's knowledge of the illness. Even without symptoms, he is now suffering severely.

Suffering—and the way in which it is confronted—is part of the fabric of human life. Part of the hospital's task should be to help the patient confront it adeptly.

. . .

Hospitals are very complex environments. In fact, it's necessary to look at three very different psycho-philosophies (the aforementioned blurring of psychology with philosophy) in order to understand them: those of the caregivers, the patients, and the organizations themselves. All three can have opposing perceptions and forces which can put them at odds with each other—and they often do.

Let's look first at the psycho-philosophy of the caregivers, since modern health care currently revolves more around them than around the patients. An important element within this is the need for the caregivers to be cared for themselves. If you could observe the conversations of medical personnel long enough during the day's activity, you would note that a great deal of attention is given to their own self-care and mutual support. An argument could be made that the emotionally draining nature of the work requires such self-attention, but I feel this is an inadequate explanation. "Burnout" is sometimes legitimate; but often is just a convenient term obscuring problems of the individual unrelated to work.

Other important elements of the caregivers' psycho-philosophy are their conflicts and feelings of undervaluation. For example, nurses serve many masters. In addition to themselves, they serve their supervisor, the patient, the patient's family, the institution, as well as the physicians. Nurses often suffer the consequences when these factions come into conflict. Not surprisingly, they can feel under-valued for their work and their strife.

As a simple example, consider Carol, a nurse who is nearing the conclusion of a double shift required because of inadequate staffing. After 16 hours, she feels so tired that her main goal is to attend to her own needs. Still, patients wish to have their own needs attended to: To ask questions, be given water, receive pain medications. Her supervisor has a reported incident to discuss. The doctors want assistance. Families want information. The institution wants Carol to focus on paperwork—while paying her less than she feels is deserved. The demands never seem to cease.

. . .

Hospitals have the same driving forces as any other organization. One force is that organizations—like people—have an instinct for survival. This may even take precedence over the hospital's successful accomplishment of its stated mission. For example, a hospital might be driven to protect its own continued existence even if a merger with another facility would serve the community more effectively. Or, for prestige or income, a facility might offer specialized services that it is ill-prepared to safely deliver.

Another force is that organizations are adaptable. If hospitals can't sell health care locally, they will sell health care education, professional conferences, administrative expertise to other organizations, training, or even colonize other communities by building outlying facilities.

Probably the most important aspect of hospitals' psycho-philosophies is that their organizations are made up of individuals. And those individuals may well put their own interests ahead of the organization's stated mission. What is best for the career of a department head or a CEO may not be best for the institution. The institution doesn't always win out. In fact, if you were to ask staff and administrators to summarize the hospital's mission statement, let alone act upon it, many would come up with only the merest approximations.

. . .

At the bottom of the pecking order is you, the patient. It's true that many hospitals do make an effort to be considerate. But patients are often little recognized except for the fact that they are requirements for the other participants to achieve their own goals. Without patients, the hospital obviously would cease to exist; and without patients, the caregivers would lose their jobs and prestige.

A main characteristic of patients is how the negative aspects of the spectrum of human concerns become intensified within them. (See Appendix A, for those interested in details.) That is, when faced with a serious or life-threatening illness, patients may feel more alone and isolated, less in control, more ignorant, and more vulnerable or mortal. These can all be felt with an intensity which virtually overwhelms them and adds to their suffering.

The hospital is ill-prepared to deal with patients' distressing feelings. In fact, a hospital tends to reinforce them. Hospitalization is a psychologically regressive experience. Patients are treated—in many ways—as if they were ignorant and helpless children to be seen and not heard, whose very companionship (visitors) is routinely regulated.

Increased feelings of isolation and mortality lead to fear. And why wouldn't the patient be frightened? He or she has been placed in a incomprehensible and uncomfortable environment, removed from both the familiar and reassuring aspects of routine daily life. All the while, the unknown looms ahead.

. . .

At their finest, hospitals are superb institutions. They proclaim a mission of care. To accomplish this care, they gather diverse and skilled professionals who are armed with modern technology. And, rarely do patients need trouble themselves with regard to the cost of all of this—at least not at the time of delivery of the services.

Unfortunately, reality sometimes lags behind idealism. The hospital's mission is often evident on paper only. The direct-care staff may be undertrained for their tasks—and so overworked—that accomplishing a care-giving mission can be difficult or impossible. And the assistance of technology can just as easily subvert care as it can enhance the stated mission. It cannot only replace the patient as the focus of attention, but can then turn upon the patient, actually causing further harm. Sophisticated diagnostic studies, such as amniocentesis, are not without their risks.

At the end of a paper-trail of admirable policies and procedures is often a paper tiger: An impotent administration unable to rid its facility of incompetent—even dangerous—doctors. Hospitals are one of the most important lines of defense for patients. Physicians applying for staff privileges need to be adequately screened. This procedure is often ineffective. Once admitted to the staff, bad doctors are frequently there to stay.

There is often an attitude of smugness and invulnerability on the part of these institutions. Sometimes this can develop because they have been fixtures in the community for many years. The fact that hospitals have largely become self-contained communities also contributes. They have lives of their own. Within their ever-expanding buildings (these days sometimes referred to as "campuses") are virtual cities containing restaurants, shops, postal facilities, security forces, laundries, educational programs—even athletic facilities. If the hospital can't grow by adding more beds, it may try to grow by merging with another facility.

In a way, the hospital administrator is more like a mayor. This sort of arrangement fosters a feeling of territoriality: A focusing and narrowing of one's own perspective onto a very small environment which becomes all-important. We all experience this in our daily lives—it is a normal phenomenon. Expressions such as "his work is his whole life" exemplify it. Unfortunately, territoriality narrows the view of the hospital, often resulting in it putting its own best interest above that of the community's.

The financial bottom line is almost as important to hospitals as it is to full-fledged businesses. In fact, you would be reasonably correct if you substituted the phrase "this business" every time you saw or heard the word "hospital." This isn't to criticize fiscal responsibility; it is only to point out its reality and raise the question of priorities.

. . .

Three major organizational tracks of a hospital—administration, physicians, and non-physician caregivers such as nurses and aides—may try to avoid interacting with each other except as absolutely necessary. Within the larger culture of the hospital, each runs its own little world. Efforts to break down the walls through such programs as TQM (Total Quality Management) have largely been failures. While we call hospitals "organizations," they are rather loosely put together. "Disorganizations" might be a more fitting term ("*dys*organizations" would provide a more medical flavor).

The situation has become so out-of-hand that hospitals generate reams of paperwork in an effort to stay even marginally in touch with and attached to their parts. The paperwork can have the effect of doing nothing more than generating further work and separation.

Only after all the segments of the organization have taken care of their own needs, do patient concerns more fully become the primary focuses of attention. Only when the individual members of the organization are reasonably comfortable, and when their collective security is assured, do they turn with greater vigor to their patients.

. . .

After being admitted to a hospital, patients begin a journey through a confusing but fairly standard maze. The hospital establishes a routine for patients, any divergence from which is seen as disruptive.

Patients may be asked to sign all manner of forms. While the spoken request is "read these and sign them," the unspoken message is often "just sign them, never mind either reading or understanding them—that would slow us down too much."

The day's routine is set up largely for the convenience of the staff. If patients balk at what they are told to do, they are perceived as non-compliant or "bad" patients or perhaps even mentally ill. Patients who are seen as overly inquisitive or non-compliant in the treatment program may even find themselves scheduled for a consultation with the psychiatrist.

When the patient representative comes around to visit, remember that the representative is likely to be an employee of the hospital. In my opinion, you run the risk of becoming the loser as the representative tries to serve two masters: patient and institution. This caution is not intended to dissuade the use of the services of a patient representative: Patients need all the help they can get. But be aware who is providing that help and who is paying the salary.

Much of the humanity of hospitals seems to be slipping away. People who were formerly called "supervising nurses" are now sometimes referred to as "managers." Care is provided by "the team." While individual staff members may maintain a personal professionalism, the aura of a healing environment seems diminished.

Hospitals often don't work for the patient because they are not set up for him or her. They are set up for the administrators, the physicians, and the other caregivers. Many hospitals are for profit, so they are largely set up to respond to the needs of owners. These people may not be even remotely connected to the community.

The only hints of "caring" in hospitals may come from (1) their marketing departments and (2) the nursing staff. The marketers will put out glossy brochures indicating that this hospital is for you and is ready to offer you the ultimate in TLC combined with modern technology. The staff may wear buttons with slogans proclaiming their caring concern for the patient. It has always seemed to me that if staff actually had this care and concern they wouldn't need buttons to proclaim it. Fortunately for us, many staff *are* concerned—buttons or not.

. . .

I don't wish to engender overly apprehensive feelings in patients entering a hospital. Hospitals are quite capable of providing concerned, high-quality, cutting-edge care. However, they may need a lot of input from the patient or family to actually deliver these goals to the individual.

Keeping in mind a few additional points may help. Those who play the largest role in actually protecting your life in the hospital may not be doctors, but nurses and aides. And these people may be too overworked (and occasionally undertrained) to save the day. Still, it helps to have the proverbial "dedicated physician" on your side.

Concerned patients and their families need to get beyond the hospitals' impressive facades, the confusing language, and the attitude of "don't ask, you wouldn't understand." In spite of all their deficiencies, they usually will function at least satisfactorily for you. But they will fail often enough to be of true concern.

Once again, the idea here is get involved. Hospitals say that they are set up for you and wish to serve you. Wouldn't it be nice if they meant what they said. Insist on it!

CHAPTER 5

Understanding Patients and Their Families

Pearl:
The patients—not the professionals—should be at the center of health care.

One of the biggest challenges of modern life is being a patient. Being a family member of a seriously ill patient is close behind it. Perhaps not surprisingly, the word "patient" is derived from the Latin term for "suffer."

Rarely do patients or families have the necessary knowledge and skills for interacting with the medical world—until it is too late to make a significant difference. Even though health care is an issue deserving of the same preparation as careers and marriage, it seldom gets the same degree of attention.

The individual should be at the center of health care—not the system. Partnerships ideally should develop primarily between the patient and the caregivers, not between the patient and the system. Within those partnerships, the issue is not, "I have a problem—what are you going to do about it?" Rather, it should be,

"How can we work together to resolve this?" A quality patient-doctor relationship can be the most powerful antidote for some patients' suffering.

. . .

The sick (and their families) are thrown into a world not of their making. Their involvement within it can be accompanied by feelings of vulnerability along with additional financial, emotional, or physical limitations. Health care is a world as unique as military life or work life, but without the accompanying training for success. Patients are, in effect, "refugees" in the medical world. Unlike the caregivers who exist within this enigmatic world, patients have no home base to call their own after they enter. They are on someone else's turf.

The system is generally not patient-centered. Its day-to-day operation is designed largely for the convenience of the medical community. It may also be inefficient, ineffective, expensive, uncomfortable, and sometimes unnecessarily dangerous. No wonder people are angry over their health care. They should be!

Despite these negative aspects, patients often have faith in their doctor and in the system, largely because they must. What choice do they have? They don't understand the illness, nor can they cure it. And they often don't even understand much of the technical language which is spoken. So, the patients must participate in their care in a fairly primitive way. He or she operates on the very basic levels of fear and survival. Perceptions involving relationships, understanding, and involvement move toward isolation, ignorance, and passivity respectively.

It's somewhat amazing how patients are caught so off guard. This patient status—be it as a surgical, medical, or psychiatric patient—is one which will befall most of us at some point in our lives. You would think we would be better prepared for what is virtually the inevitable. Still, few people are prepared for their involvement in this complex system.

. . .

Patients are not a homogeneous group. Some people have special needs peculiar to their own lives and illnesses, while there are others who do share common problems. For example, children have unique problems and require help due to their obvious limitations in dealing with the medical establishment. Like other patients, they are sometimes subject to harmful and unnecessary treatment, including unnecessary surgeries and inappropriate psychiatric hospitalization and/or medication to control behaviors. There must be someone to speak for them.

However, children's greatest health problem may be their parents or guardians. These adults may fail to provide the opportunity for basic medical care which is available to their charges. Failure to get immunizations is perhaps the best example. Additionally, parents often provide negative role-modeling (by smoking or excessive drinking), while not providing adequate positive input (discussing health care issues at home, engaging in personal exercise programs, and so on). Children need mature adults to apply the "Four Steps to Better Care" on their behalf.

The elderly are often overmedicated and undercared for. In fact, successful treatment of elderly patients often begins with the recognition of the excessive prescription medications some take. Often the elderly need someone to advocate for them due to physical or mental incapacities. Perhaps more so than with any other group, the medical profession adopts a paternalistic "we know what's best for you" attitude toward them. There is often no one to challenge this.

Another group that needs special attention are the mentally ill, who are often warehoused rather than treated. Of all types of illnesses, emotional disorders are probably least understood. Care for psychiatric patients must be given against a complex legal background, which even practitioners and attorneys don't always understand or agree upon. And all this doesn't even begin to address the issue of the stigma of psychiatric impairment which serves to further isolate patients.

The physically challenged are also subject to an infantilization and patronizing attitude from the medical profession. Too often, they are seen for their weaknesses rather than for their strengths. Their existing physical limitations can confound treatment for other problems. For instance, being wheelchair-bound makes exercise more difficult in controlling obesity.

Women, an even larger group, have a long history of abuse at the hands of the medical system. These problems range all the way from frank sexual abuse by "caregivers," to assaults because of unnecessary surgery, to more subtle situations such as patronizing attitudes and misdiagnosis due to sexual stereotyping. (A number of books, such as *The New Our Bodies, Ourselves* [1992] give the kind of attention to some of these issues which I could not hope to match in this work.)

I've named just a few groups here. But whether patients are from within the general population or from within one of these special groups, they need to be heard and responded to as individuals. They are not "the gallbladder," "the Alzheimer's," "the manic," "the hip fracture," "the stroke," or "the kid."

Educational organizations, support groups, and/or advocacy assistance are available to patients or families dealing with a variety of health problems. Among these are migraine headaches, Crohn's disease, the late effects of polio, manic-depressive illness (now called "bipolar"), obesity, Alzheimer's disease, cancer, and many, many more. If you're dealing with a serious illness, the chances are excellent that there is an organization for you. Your doctor, local public or medical library, or the National Self-Help Clearinghouse in New York City at 25 West 43rd Street; New York, NY 10036 are among some of the many sources of potential information.

To whatever extent possible, people need to understand their own situation and be their own best advocates. Ideally, the medical profession should at least take note of the efforts and programs put forth by patient organizations.

. . .

Patients face a number of significant obstacles in obtaining adequate care. One of the most serious is being identified with a label rather than being seen for the suffering individuals that they are. Not only does this result in depersonalization, but it interferes with treatment. For example, instead of being Mrs. Smith, the patient with diabetes, Mrs. Smith simply becomes "the diabetic." The implication is that to know her label is to know both Mrs. Smith and her illness. Of course, this is not true.

Other significant problems include the patient being perceived as an income source, an inconvenience, or an irritation. While there are, indeed, obnoxious people who get ill and become patients, many patients are perceived as irritations in the path of the doctor's life simply because of the nature of their illnesses or the additional professional burdens placed upon the physician who already sees himself or herself as overworked.

Patients can develop strategies for countering these negative factors. One tool is to follow the "Four Steps to Better Care:"

1. *Understanding* of your clinical situation and the health care delivery system—as well as understanding yourself and your caregivers.

2. Having active and full *involvement* in your care—if necessary, insisting upon it.

3. Accepting your own personal *responsibility*.

4. Recognizing your *authority* in speaking up, in exploring options, and in making many ultimate decisions.

Having an approach for acquiring reasonable clinical knowledge, as well as information on health care delivery, is essential to carry out these steps. Here are a few resources:

- A personal medical reference library (see Chapter 23). If you have a computer and a modem, you have access to even more information on-line.
- Librarians in both public and medical libraries can assist you in obtaining books and articles and by doing searches of topics. Especially utilize the directories in the reference sections of medical libraries.
- Ask physicians and other professionals for references dealing with specific problems.
- Pharmaceutical companies often provide literature related to their products. Write or call them.
- There may be patient support or information organizations which can help.
- Ask anyone—friends, other patients, insurance agents, co-workers—whoever you think might know something about your problem or know of resources. (But don't just accept anyone's information at face value.)

Throughout this book, I'll frequently mention your need for information. Since we are living in the Information Age, most questions shouldn't have to remain unanswered. Fire up your computer, go down to the library, get on the phone, visit facilities, pick up literature, write to agencies and organizations. Be creative and energetic in gathering knowledge which will be in your best interest and that of your family. Ask! Be assertive! There's lots of help out there.

All these practical approaches for becoming informed are still not adequate for successful "patienthood." People who have developed a satisfying philosophy of life—that is, they have an understanding of the meaning of their existence—will suffer less during a period of illness. Other assistance might come from one's personal faith or religious community.

People may need all the help they can get. Witnessing a loss of control over their own bodies and lives, they may experience regrets over past mistakes or losses. All these can add to the patient's suffering. For some, serious illness actually provides a positive turning point in their lives. It forces them to do what we all should be attempting prior to a devastating illness: sorting out lives, goals and priorities—and enjoying to the fullest those blessings which we do have.

Patients can share feelings, thoughts, and even suffering with family, friends, and professionals. But, some things, such as the actual experience of pain, must be borne alone. Even if we should die surrounded by those we love, we will still make this ultimate journey alone.

. . .

Fortunate is the patient who has support of family and friends to share the burden and suffering of illness. But those closest to the patient often feel as helpless as the patient. "I don't know what to do," or "I don't know what to say" are common responses.

The simplest solution for family and friends is to acknowledge to both themselves and to the patient the realities of the illness as well as the realities of their concern and love. This can be in an honest, direct, but compassionate and—where appropriate—hopeful fashion. But it must always be done with an appreciation of where the patient is at emotionally and intellectually in dealing with the illness. If the patient is not ready for active involvement by others, then family and friends may need to hold back.

The family can play a strong positive role in opening the door to conversation, practical issues, and appropriate requests. When the time is right, they can ask, "Is there anything I can do for you?" or "Is there anything that you would like to talk about?"

Somewhat more direct is, "Are there plans or tasks I can help you with?" If all of these still seem too intrusive, simply a presence and a willingness to continue topics introduced by the patient can be very productive.

Just as is the case with patients, the personal philosophies and faith of family and friends can be pillars of strength in meeting their own emotional needs at this time. They can lean on—and share thoughts with—each other for mutual benefit. They can also seek out specific support organizations which may deal with the illness.

The medical profession should not deny patients and families access to each other during times of a health crisis unless absolutely necessary for care. Even giving a patient access to his or her pets as the circumstances allow should not be overlooked as a valuable source of great comfort.

In spite of having great potential as a positive force, family involvement can be a mixed blessing, especially if there are pre-existing problems within the family. Both patients and family must realize that an illness, in itself, will not set everything right. This is not Hollywood. There may not be the strength within the patient to deal with long-festering problems. If indicated, the doctor or hospital staff can assist in getting help with such issues.

Families will often act in what they see as the best interest of the patient, but their efforts may grow out of guilt rather than love or concern. Doctors often hear that "money is no object" and "we want to know that we did everything that could be done." But what about the patient? He or she may not desire the prolonged suffering and efforts such actions would bring.

It becomes a heavy burden on the family to pick up the mantle of responsibility when the patient is no longer able to handle it. Ideally, their strength and energy will remain long after it is depleted in the patient. But, families must appreciate their limits. They cannot make everything better. They cannot prevent suffering. And their own lives must go on.

Ideally, patients will have paved the way for smoother decision-making by providing, in advance, a durable power of attorney for health care and/or a living will. These documents, which might be provided by an attorney or hospital, can give guidelines for the family to follow in a time of crisis and decision-making. But as long as the patient is capable of doing so, he or she must be included in all appropriate communications and choices.

Families should not be overzealous in speaking for the patient. Even the very ill should be allowed to do and say what he or she properly can. As a practitioner, one of the most frustrating and unproductive tasks I get involved in is when family members unnecessarily become intermediaries in relaying information. Often these patients are quite capable of giving me better information directly.

As necessary, family and friends must become the eyes, ears, voice, and even protector of the patient. Ideally, extremely ill patients should not be left alone in a hospital setting. This may not make the staff happy, but families should be as assertive as possible. They can request the physician's cooperation in planning the family's presence.

. . .

Our society can't afford to lose the energy, responsibility, vested interest, and creativity of individuals as positive forces in their own care. Nor can we afford to lose the compassion and innovation which ordinary people can collectively contribute to our nation's efforts in delivering better care to all citizens.

At the most crucial times of illness, the high technology of modern medicine may become dwarfed in importance by the high touch of family and loved ones. Laying on of the hands isn't just for the clergy or physicians. All those who love and are loved by the patient can affect his or her care deeply.

CHAPTER 6

Understanding Nurses

Pearl:

If the nursing profession was free to reach its full potential, health care would improve 100 percent.

Nurses may have *the* most rewarding—and difficult—job of any health care professional. They may also have what is the most rapidly changing role in health care delivery.

An argument could be made that nursing represents the very epitome of the caring professions: Nurses are the most "hands on," selfless, and available of all the healers. They are the last person many of us will ever see on earth. In spite of this, they are markedly less financially rewarded and often less valued than physicians.

A few years ago I would have also suggested that nurses were perhaps more satisfied in their work than other health care professionals. But today's nurses are embattled souls. While their calling is special, their profession may be headed for serious problems for a number of reasons. One thing which appears certain at this time is that their role—for better or for worse—will continue to expand.

(While recognizing the increasingly important role men play in nursing, for simplicity in this chapter, I'll refer to nurses as "she." Currently, the great majority are women.)

Once a physician prescribes treatment, often it is only the nurse who stands between the patient and disaster. This is true regardless of the correctness of the treatment plan. The nurse's potential to institute and carry out harmful and self-serving approaches on her own initiative is much less than it is for doctors.

The psychology of the nurse is complex. Of course, nurses share the same basic needs and emotions of us all. But the nature of their profession—and the recent profound changes in it—complicates the task of fully understanding nursing. Today, a dark side can be seen in the psycho-philosophy of nursing which surely drains it of some of its strengths and diminishes its effectiveness. I believe there are several reasons this has evolved:

1. Many nurses have moved from the bedside to the corporate desk. While there is nothing inherently wrong with this, these nurses often find themselves moving into a business environment which is foreign to their training. Additionally, this new setting also has its own serious set of problems. Nurses undergo a difficult transition from being healers to joining those who share the corporate concern for the bottom line. The new work may seem to them incompatible with their original goals.

   Even within the hospital setting, nurses have become "de-medicalized." What used to be called a "nursing supervisor" may now be a "manager" or "resource person." Those nurses still working at the bedside have less and less of an opportunity to relate to—and comfort—their patients. Older nurses who fondly recall the (not entirely) "good old days" may be more dissatisfied than their younger colleagues who know only modern nursing.

2. Many people enter nursing with an unconscious desire to resolve their own problems or to get relief for their own psychological needs. The result is an emphasis on self, moving the nurse away from the patient. (Much the same could be said for physicians and other caregivers.)

3. Nurses who remain at the bedside are caught between the proverbial rock and a hard place: They have much responsibility but little authority. When they battle with physicians over the appropriateness of patient care, nurses are almost never the victors. They must reconcile their orders with their conscience. (Nurses are employees of the hospital and directly responsible to it, *not* to the physicians. However, most hospitals will not risk alienating their physicians in disputes between doctor and nurse.)

4. As with other under-recognized people in our society who perform important and difficult tasks, we fail to give nurses their just due—both in terms of prestige or pay. Certainly, part of this is a gender equality issue.

5. While generally well-educated, nurses are often still under-trained for some of their assigned tasks. Although they may have advanced training as nurse practitioners, nurses are nevertheless far removed from the knowledge of practicing physicians. Regrettably, they are too often called upon to stand inappropriately in his or her place. In some instances, nurses are asked to over-reach with

regard to providing certain kinds of education to patients, being front-line responders to complex critical emergency situations, fielding patient inquiries over the phone, or even prescribing medicines. I'm well aware of the argument that nurse practitioners work out of their own special background and are not "junior physicians." But in reality, the latter is what often occurs. In this era of blurring roles between nurses and other professionals, it's time for a careful re-evaluation of definitions. What is a nurse? What is a doctor?

. . .

What moves people to enter nursing rather than other careers? As the modern medical world continues to change rapidly, so will the answers to this question. I think that four specific reasons currently stand out: idealism, practicality, sexual inequality, and new opportunities.

- Idealism is a powerful force: Good people still wish to do good things. Nursing is a field which holds tremendous potential for those who wish to help other human beings.
- The practicality of nursing appeals to many women (and increasingly, to many men as well). Many young people wish to have a career which will well serve their community. They may also wish to have a family. Nursing is seen as a compatible choice for both needs: It usually does not require extremely long periods of preparation, it can provide flexible hours conducive to family life, and is a field which can be moved in and out of throughout life depending on the family situation.
- As much as we might want it to disappear, sexual inequality still exists. Since nursing is still seen as a more

available career path for women, many take that route.

- The increasing availability of corporate roles, and the opportunities for expanded clinical roles, are becoming additional factors in the decision to select nursing. Nurses can use their basic clinical training as a springboard to a number of career tracks. Some of their options are:
  - — Traditional hospital and office roles.
  - — Clinical nursing outside these two settings (in schools, work places, public health).
  - — Extended roles, e.g., anesthetists, clinical nurse specialists, nurse practitioners, midwives.
  - — Administrative and business opportunities for nurses are available. Working for companies involved in managed care allows them to use their nursing knowledge away from the bedside.

Nurses have varying qualifications. An RN (registered nurse) may or may not have been trained in the context of a bachelor's degree program. Either way, she must pass a qualifying exam prior to registration. LPN's (Licensed Practical Nurses) are less trained and are licensed with more limitations than RN's. In addition, there are clinical nurse specialists, nurse practitioners, nurse midwives, and nurse anesthetists. All have additional training. And although we do speak of "nurses training," one might legitimately raise the question of whether nurses are "trained" or "educated."

Probably the most prevalent image of a nurse within a hospital setting is that of the "med-surg" nurse. This is the general duty nurse who is likely to be seen on many hospital floors (and in soap operas). But nurses can also focus their training for such areas as the intensive care unit, emergency room, pediatric and obstetrical departments, operating room, and in administrative or supervisory positions.

If the work of anyone can appropriately be described as diversified, it is that of a general duty hospital nurse. Part of this diversity comes from the fact that these nurses work in a very complex environment, serving many masters. Their patients may see them as competent professionals and empathetic listeners. However, direct hands-on work may be a relatively small proportion of their day's work.

To the family of a patient, the nurse is often counselor, educator, and information source. To the doctor, the nurse may be seen as both helper and surrogate. To the administration of the hospital, she is risk manager and provider of statistical input. At other times, she's transporter of patients, housekeeper, secretary, lab technician, and supporter of co-workers. She is usually a dynamo. Whatever else you may consider a general duty nurse, you can rarely consider her as lazy or as having a cushy job.

The work is definitely less glamorous or heroic than that of physicians. While their work provides continuing life-lines for the patients, their efforts are frequently undervalued by patient and doctor as well as society in general. Although nurses are responsible for literally *giving* the shots, they rarely have the opportunity to *call* them.

Nurses who have both the time and the concern can incorporate the marvelous gift of listening into patient care. Many hospitalized patients consider themselves fortunate if they can spend a few minutes a day with a doctor, often responding to pointed, focused questions by him or her. The nurse who can sit by the bedside, listening to the patient who is dealing with suffering, achieves some of the most fulfilling moments of any caregiver. But as the roles of nurses change and expand, will TLC become less of a defining characteristic?

. . .

A nurse's day typically begins with "report" to each other. This is the main organizing activity in the shift when duties are assigned and plans are made. At this time, the nurses from the preceding shift will pass on the relevant clinical information to the nurses coming on duty. Information is exchanged on new admissions to the floor, planned discharges, and significant changes in the medical status and treatment programs of current patients. The report previously was typically "live," but in recent years, audiotaping the report for the next shift has become popular.

Poor communications skills, tardiness, interruptions, work overload, and lack of focus can all contribute to a less than adequate report. That's unfortunate, because report is truly a critical task. Complicating report is the additional (and sometimes inadequate) effort to bring up to speed nurses who are borrowed from other areas of the hospital or who work part-time.

Following report, nurses may make their own rounds, going from room to room and physically checking on each patient. They, or the nurses' aides, will also take "vitals" as time permits. This involves checking the patient's blood pressure, pulse, respirations, and temperature. Morning nursing rounds provide an opportunity for patients to find out what's on their agenda for the day, as well as when the doctor might be in. Patients can also convey any new questions or concerns to the nurses during rounds.

Patients should learn the names of their nurses, and be sure the nurses know them by face and name. It's probably wishful thinking on my part that nurses will call the patient "Ms. Jones" or "Mr. Jones" and introduce themselves as "Ms. Smith" or "Ms. Johnson," but it sure would be a nice professional touch. I know the response of the profession is that patients like the informality. When I'm a patient, I like the professionalism of formal titles.

Doctors arriving on the floor may stop and ask for a report from the nurse. Unfortunately, this isn't always the case, and valuable information often goes uncommunicated. Sometimes nurses accompany the doctor on his or her rounds and assist with a variety of procedures such as dressing changes or suture removal (nurses often do these tasks independently). To the detriment of everyone, nurses are often too busy to adequately provide such services to either patients or doctors. Some tasks simply get done suboptimally.

Since families have more access to the nursing staff than they have to physicians, they will often turn to the nurses as their primary source of information as well as comfort. Nurses can provide useful information regarding the general status of the patient, as well as occasional specifics. Unfortunately, nurses sometimes have less of a grasp of the basic illness and the prognosis than you might suspect. Long chats with the nurse, regardless of how informative they may be, should not routinely take the place of input from the physician to patient and/or family.

"Charting" is another time-consuming, but necessary task for nurses. All relevant nursing information must be included in the patient's clinical record in adequate detail. If done appropriately, charting becomes a valuable clinical tool for both monitoring the patient's progress as well as for providing useful information to other staff. Generally, nurses' handwriting is fairly good (definitely better on average than physicians'). But, when they occur, illegible notes are worse than useless. They consume valuable time while provide no help, and can even cause confusion. Much of charting is done for purely legal reasons, documenting the information which the hospital attorneys will want to see in case of a lawsuit. (Nurses' notes on the chart can also provide a source of humor due to their abbreviated format. For instance, a reader might be informed that "Doctor here. Had good bowel movement.")

Closely related to charting is the issue of confidentiality. What goes into your record will be there for years, and it will be available to many eyes. If there is material which you, as a patient, feel you do not wish to have charted, discuss this with the doctor or the nurse as appropriate.

Nurses also "pass meds" to patients several times a day. While nurses always try to see that each patient takes exactly what medicine was prescribed, it is certainly appropriate for patients to question any medication that appears different or unusual. And patients should know the purpose of each medication. Mistakes—sometimes extremely serious ones—can be made when a physicians' sloppy writing causes the nurse to bring the wrong medication.

Some, but not all, nurses will start I.V.'s. Unfortunately, the general nursing staff is at times poorly skilled in this procedure. There are almost always people potentially available who are more accomplished. Patients shouldn't allow themselves to be stuck repeatedly without asking for someone else to perform the task. Much the same can be said about obtaining blood for laboratory tests. Speak up to get the most skilled person available if there is no success with the first or second attempt.

Throughout the day, nurses may be called upon to perform one of the most critical functions of hospital care: admitting and discharging patients. These activities set the stage for successful hospital stays, as well as carrying over into the post-hospital period.

It is usually the nurse, not the doctor, who is first involved with the patient after arrival on the hospital floor. The information the nurse gathers is part of the foundation for subsequent care. The patient should not only cooperate as fully as possible, but even take the initiative to improve the quality of the information received by the nurse since the physician may be making critical decisions based on this data.

The time of discharge can be as critical an event as the time of admission. This is the opportunity to bring together all the loose ends and unresolved issues. It's also a chance for the patient to evaluate the hospital stay: "Did I get the relief or services for which I came?"

While much of the discharge process must be personally handled by the physician, it's usually the nurses who provide much of the instructional information to the patient based on orders by the physicians. (More on this process can be found in Chapter 11.)

Patients being discharged must make sure that they understand clearly the information the nurses are relaying. The nurses will probably provide written sheets of instructions and perhaps present the patients with prescriptions from the doctors. The instructions and medications should be reviewed carefully.

If no information has been provided about follow-up appointments, question the nurses on this and/or ask them to contact the physicians for such information. The patients should always leave the hospital with the feeling that all significant issues have been not only addressed, but resolved as far as possible.

. . .

The list of nurses' responsibilities and work is almost endless. I've listed only a very few duties here. Nurses also teach patients, are often first on the scene at a "code" or emergency, give baths, make beds, pass trays, interpret patterns on monitors, supervise other staff, and provide emotional support for the patients' families. These days, there is also paperwork, paperwork, and more paperwork.

Perhaps less skilled or differently trained personnel could be doing some of these activities. However, there is much to be said for the patient contact which many of these tasks provide, as well as how they enhance the continuity of care.

Many of the nurses' responsibilities center at the "nurses' station." Excessive time spent here is time away from patients. Certainly some necessary work needs to be done at the nurses' station: charting, setting up medications, and so on. But when the station is understaffed, nurses' time is wasted here on answering phones and doing unnecessary paperwork. Nurses often find themselves substituting for less extensively trained—but extremely valuable—ward clerks or secretaries.

While nurses almost always work very hard, there are periods when socializing with other staff seems to come first. This is especially true on psychiatric units. There, one often hears extremely involved discussions of administrative issues not at all critical for the moment. Or personal issues will consume huge blocks of time.

Even though some of this "wasted" time is probably a necessary response to the tremendous pressures felt by nurses, it makes them less available to both patients and the medical staff. Nurses need to have enough help so that they can take necessary breaks and be involved in such discussions in more private settings and at more convenient times. Unlike other workers, they're not simply inconveniencing customers—they're interrupting potentially critical tasks.

Before leaving the nurse's routine, it would be appropriate to comment on current trends in nursing attire. Traditional medical uniforms provided a marvelously potent and even healing symbol. For the very confused patient they also provided a mental anchor for basic recognition of staff. For those patients who are more mentally competent than this, appropriate uniforms would still be an assistance considering the vast array of personnel that one now sees on a hospital floor. (It's only fair to report that my wife, Pat—the nurse—strongly disagrees with my view on nurse's uniforms. Am I being too theoretical and not practical enough?)

All manner, color and combinations of clothing is seen. The worst is on some psychiatric units where it is difficult to even tell the patients from the staff. In fact, I have often seen patients on these units more appropriately dressed and appearing more professional than the staff.

Another issue of dress is the frequent occurrence of people, including nurses, wearing hospital "greens" at the shopping mall, in the food store, and in other non-clinical settings. I wonder how many people so attired are actually health care workers. Part of the purpose of this clothing is to assure safe and sanitary attire. I am not much of a fan of whatever "fashion statement" this clothing is making in public.

. . .

The above "snapshot" of the nurses' routine misses much of the complexity of the profession—a profession upon which will ultimately rest the destinies of many of us.

The trend in medicine has been to admit fewer, but more seriously ill, patients and to have them in the hospital for briefer periods of time. That is, the acuity, or the "quality" of their illness, if you will, has gone up. In spite of this change, nurses' complaints of having to care for too many patients often fall on deaf ears. Administrators may parade statistics that show they are not taking care of any more patients than they were 10 or 15 years ago, but this ignores the fact that nurses must now deal with a sicker population. As if just caring for more severely ill patients isn't enough, nurses must also deal with the pressure of meeting the demands of their many bosses and dealing with an unending flow of paperwork. In the midst of all this, nurses have their own conflicted feelings to confront.

These feelings may involve carrying out physicians' orders which they may question. Unlike physicians who can largely focus on their work (often thanks to stay-at-home spouses), nurses often find themselves combining work with concerns of their own children, household management, and day-to-day finances.

Nurses are often asked to "float." This means going to other floors which may be even more understaffed than their own and helping out for a period of time. Nurses often have strong feelings when they are "pulled" to work in these other settings. They are often not trained for these areas and feel uncomfortable or even unethical in trying to adequately care for patients there.

When staff call in ill, the nurses may be asked to work a "double"—that is, a double shift. This causes complications for patients and staff: the intensity of the work is too great to be able to focus on it productively for such an extended period of time, and care is diminished.

. . .

A nurse's relationship with a patient is at the crux of the profession. It's largely why many nurses went into training in the first place. Nurses would like to be able to spend time with the patients and bring comfort, but hospital administration and staffing patterns may hinder these efforts.

Not all patients and all nurses are compatible with each other. Both must learn to ignore, or (more ideally) confront, personality frictions so that they can reach beyond these to the important mutual task of dealing with the patient's suffering. And, like everyone, nurses have "bad days." Unfortunately, the medical profession usually offers little support to help our nursing staffs during these times.

Conflicts sometimes arise between patients and nurses over patients' request for medications. The patients should know what medicines are available "PRN" (which means "as needed"). Patients should be frank in making their physical discomforts and emotional uneasiness known to the nurses. Nurses and patients need to have clear lines of understanding about the use of the available medications in these situations. Patients should not feel guilty—or be made to feel guilty by the staff—if they make reasonable requests for medications. They are not "wimps" because they are legitimately in pain or have some other distressing symptom.

If the nurses don't make themselves available to the family, the family should take the initiative in asking for time to sit down and discuss the patient's care. Families need to understand that nurses are bound by confidentiality regarding information about patients. As much as they may wish to share some information, they may not have the patient's permission. Families shouldn't push nurses for material to which they are not legally entitled. Fortunately, permission is usually easily obtained from the patient. However, the bottom line is that competent patients are the ones to decide what information is to be shared with anyone.

In the relationship between patients and nurses, it is true that "action speaks louder than words." Nurses who work hard to make time to be at the bedside demonstrate a greater commitment to care than all the slick marketing brochures in the world.

On the other hand, patients shouldn't abuse care. They should not desire, nor allow themselves, to be infantilized by nursing staff. They should appropriately demonstrate to the nurses what they are capable of and be self-sufficient to whatever extent is possible and reasonable. The extent of patient self-care needs to be carefully worked out between patient, doctor, and nurse.

The nurse's relationship with the doctor is the stuff of soap operas. It has all the required ingredients: excitement, fascination, anger, triumph, and dramatic action. For better or for worse, it may at times even have romance and sex.

At their best, the relationships between doctors and nurses are marvelously productive and professional ones. Nurses are present 24 hours a day as compared to the physician, whose time there is limited. They can report helpful information to which the physicians may never be privy. The skills of the physician and nurse at the bedside compliment each other. And the solidarity shown between them can be a healing force for the patient.

On the negative side, the relationship between physician and nurse can be quite contentious. Many doctors certainly don't see the nurse as an equal. There can be misconceptions on both sides. Physicians often undervalue the work of nurses. But, without the nurse's help, a doctor's work would be virtually impossible. In spite of this, doctors are often arrogant toward them. Physicians' medical training has portrayed the nurse as their handmaiden.

Nurses, on the other hand, often do not have an appreciation for the years of training physicians must complete. Nurses' training is much different than that of physicians', and they cannot have the same decision-making power. There is an old platitude which is cruel but in some ways true: if nurses want to be doctors, they should go to medical school.

But nurses aren't doctors with less training: They are medical professionals with *different* training. Without significant additional training, doctors and nurses cannot substitute for each other. (In truth, it's unlikely that doctors would last for even a day trying to competently perform nursing duties.)

If we really want to relieve the physician shortage, the pool of caring nurses who might be interested in going to medical school (with an improved, shorter, and more efficient curriculum) would be a good place to start. This is a much better solution than having turf issues between doctors and nurses. I'd love to see this country have an additional 100,000 physicians who were formerly nurses. I think many nurses would choose this route if it were offered in a workable fashion.

In the meantime, I support nurses (and other health care professionals) doing physician-like work in those rural and urban areas where physicians have reneged on their collective responsibility. In fact, I support the expanded role of nurses in all ways that are appropriate. However, I would caution against confusing the essential role of the nurse with the essential role of the physician. Our lives could depend on recognizing this distinction.

The nursing profession follows the same forces (as discussed in Chapter Two) as does any other organization. It, too, sees "more" and "bigger" as better. In this case it's more autonomy, expanded roles, and bigger incomes. They also will adapt their mission in order for professional survival as they see it. This is in part why so many nurses have moved away from the bedside and toward roles previously seen as within the domain of physicians.

Part of the relationship problems between nurses and doctors arises not out of clinical decision-making issues or power struggles, but from what nurses observe of the personal qualities of physicians. Often physicians are seen as too hurried, unconcerned about the suffering of their patients, as threats to the professional egos of the nurses, and as more focused upon themselves, their images and incomes. And, often, this is true.

Nurses sometimes are so intimidated by doctors, that they avoid important communications with them. Better to let the patient's blood pressure drop a little more than wake up the doctor again tonight. It's not the physician's real or imagined power which is feared, but rather the assaults upon the nurses' psyche.

Regardless, hospitalized patients should depend not upon the doctor *or* the nurse but upon the two working as a vital team. They are two intermeshed gears in the mechanism of patients' survival and must maintain appropriate contact in a smooth-working and well-oiled environment. Medical schools would do well to have a course called "Dealing with Nurses;" nursing schools should similarly have a course called "Dealing with Doctors."

. . .

Nurses are definitely the backbone of the medical world. Without the efforts of the nurse, many of the positive aspects of modern health care couldn't be implemented. But their tasks are more than just doing procedures and passing on clinical information. Equally important are relationships, communicating, sharing, and empathy. The nurses must be able to do almost impossible tasks, not just one at a time, but simultaneously.

If patients are to receive the care they require (or that they simply desire), they must develop a finer understanding of both the role and the psycho-philosophy of nurses. Doctors would be well advised to do the same. Nurses, on the other hand, may need to reevaluate their philosophy and their psychology in light of the ever-changing pressures of modern health care.

In spite of its imperfections, patients and physicians owe much more than a tip of the hat to the nursing profession. We owe it our support and an effort to understand its work and its pressures. Patients certainly owe it something more meaningful than a box of candy or a perfunctory "thank you" at the time of discharge from the hospital. Perhaps respect and support for better treatment of nurses, would be more appreciated.

Even the best nurses need help. Patients dealing with nurses would do well to remember to implement the "Four Steps to Better Care:" (1) understanding, (2) involvement, (3) responsibility, and (4) authority.

. . .

The nursing profession is in serious trouble. It's being wounded from the inside as it deals with boundary issues. From the outside it's assaulted with unrealistic demands while being grossly undervalued.

My response, as largely put forth in this chapter, has been to suggest an understanding of the influences affecting the nursing profession—and to suggest a consideration of what constitutes the very essence of nursing. Taken separately, some of my comments may be seen as anti-feminist, anti-nursing, greedily protective of the physician's "turf," or simply reactionary. None of this is my intention. I do feel that nursing is so sacred and wonderfully unique that it should not be changed simply to accommodate a perception of providing "cheaper" care.

Nurses are special people. We are less than fair to them if we fail to make an effort to understand and support this complex and caring profession.

CHAPTER 7

Understanding the Languages of Health Care

Pearl:

Words are one of medicine's most potent instruments—and should be used with great care and expertise.

Physicians' handwriting is so notoriously illegible that for years it has been the subject of jokes. It seems as though only pharmacists have the ability to read it. Unfortunately, doctors' verbal communications can be equally uninformative.

Words should be one of the physician's most valuable tools. This is obvious in fields such as psychotherapy where talking (and listening) is raised to a high art, or when a doctor must convey clinical information to a patient. Words are also used to comfort, to teach, and even to intentionally obscure reality. But little, if any, attention is given during medical training to the skillful use of language.

The proper words can bring not only comfort, but even a cure, to patients. Words can ignite the enthusiasm of medical students and provide physicians the means for cooperation and progress with patients. But the wrong words can just as easily hinder all these efforts and thwart the healing process.

Physicians actually have a number of languages by which they communicate in their work. Most prevalent of these is common English—a language they share with patients and colleagues alike. Common as it may be, this language is often not used by physicians in a clear, informative, compassionate, and enlightening fashion.

Another language is technical in nature: A highly complex, sophisticated means of expression, not extensively understood by the laypeople. This language includes such medical terms as lupus, sarcoma, tomography, "hyper-al," and EEG. It's the physician's responsibility to provide a meaningful translation to patients when necessary.

There is also what I call a "third language"—a kind of slang—which is rarely seen in clinical writing. However, it is frequently used by the physicians in their private conversations. Carl Sandburg called slang "a language that rolls up its sleeves, spits on its hands, and goes to work." This third language can—but doesn't always—do that. Supermarket tabloids would probably call it the *secret* language of doctors. It's unfortunate that most people do not understand it because it provides some of the best insights into the physician's mind. For this reason, this least accessible language will be the primary focus of this chapter. Some of these usages may also occur outside of health care. I have primarily culled them from informal discussions over the years.

. . .

The third language may involve a single word such as "retrospectroscope" (the use of hindsight), a brief phase such as "benign neglect" (helping the patient by occasionally simply doing nothing), or a saying such as the one used to describe how students are sometimes taught procedures: "see one; do one; teach one."

In looking at these expressions, keep in mind the intimate association between what is said and the feeling behind the words.

Look at the nuances and significance of the choice of words making up this third language. Sometimes a word isn't just a word—sometimes it conveys quite accurately in its tone what doctors *really* mean.

. . .

A major use of the third language is in teaching both students and residents. Studying medicine can be boring as well as stimulating. A colorful phrase or an exciting word can be the verbal equivalent of a good 2 x 2 color slide in keeping a class alert. It can teach an important idea or aid in its retention.

Descriptions of such body products such as "currant-jelly stools," "coffee-ground emesis," and "cheesy exudate" are certainly colorful expressions, but they are in the mainstream of medicine's technical language, not part of the third language.

Students learn a valuable concept when their instructors speak of prescribing "tincture of time" or providing the patient with "benign neglect" or even "masterful neglect" (I always tell my students that *masterful* neglect is only for the additionally credentialed board certified specialists). As a former general practitioner, I've learned the wisdom of utilizing "cigar treatment" in dealing with difficult obstetrical problems—that is, to intervene quickly during a delivery, but do anything else (like smoking a cigar in the doctor's lounge) to keep from being unnecessarily meddlesome. Recalling to put in a final "husband's stitch" (a term some find offensive) is a reminder to do an adequate stitching of an episiotomy, an incision sometimes made to widen the birth canal. If a patient's problem should happen to be a "fascinoma" (a particularly fascinating medical problem), all the better for the educational interest it will generate.

Students can be made aware of the "double diagnostic" examination which occurs during the initial interview as patient and doctor evaluate or "diagnose" each other. And in talking to the patient, the interviewer communicates best by using everyday "kitchen language" instead of technical terminology. Being aware of "Monday morning flu" helps physicians recall a unique phenomenon of alcoholism (calling in sick after a weekend binge).

Some elements of the third language contain a great deal of wisdom. For example, on the orthopedic service, students might learn that "the enemy of good is better"—a reminder that too much manipulating of a fracture (efforts to "set" it) can do more harm than good. The neurologist understands that "everything is connected to everything else."

The surgeon knows that "all bleeding stops—eventually." Students and residents often write down many of these "pearls" in their "portable brains" (small notebooks to be kept in a pocket of their white coat at all times). Sometimes the information they're given is based on a "series of one" (limited personal experience) rather than on a large scientific sampling.

. . .

The third language is occasionally used for brevity and clarity. The field of surgery—in which time is of the essence—is replete with examples of the third language. Here it may be used as a form of shorthand speech.

When the surgical field becomes obscured with blood, the assistant is told to "suck" (the blood) and then perhaps to "buzz" (the bleeder). This is faster than telling the assistant to "use the negative pressure of the suction tube to remove body fluids from the field and then apply an electrical current to cause coagulation at the site of extravasation." "Suck...buzz," says it all.

If a patient has sustained multiple traumatic injuries, he or she may be described facetiously as needing a "bodygram" for further diagnosis. This entails taking a large number of "flicks" (X-rays), instead of limited views of a few specific areas. If the patient's heart stops while in the radiology department, he or she may need to be "tubed" and "bagged" (a breathing tube is inserted into the windpipe and a breathing bag used to provide adequate oxygen).

If the situation in the OR is urgent, there may need to be a "crash" induction in order to get the patient quickly anesthetized. The staff may need to do a "horrendoplasty" (a horrendous procedure) and will, therefore need to have enough equipment for lengthy and extensive surgery. An emergency room physician notes a suitcase sitting next to a patient in an examination cubicle. To him or her, this represents a "positive suitcase sign" and is an indication that this patient will be hard to avoid admitting. This suspicion is reinforced by a "positive tail-light sign" as the family registers the patient and then drives away.

. . .

Medicine and surgery can sound like very violent fields. Doctors even refer to their therapeutic tools as their "armamentarium" (strictly speaking, not a third language term). After all, patients may be "blasted" (dosed) with high doses of "poisons" (medications). When people with alcoholism get "burned out," there may not be much left of their mental well-being. Following a severe auto accident, the "orthopods" (bone doctors) do their own version of "body and fender work" (repairs). Patients "go down the tubes." Obstetricians "pit out" their patients (prescribe Pitocin) to hasten delivery, while emergency room doctors work down in "the pit" (the emergency room).

Women bleeding vaginally may have their "hysters heisted" (have a hysterectomy). An obstetrician may assist a difficult delivery by applying "blades" (forceps) to a baby's head. If urgency or circumstances demand, anesthesia may be limited to "silver bullet anesthesia" as the patient just bites down real hard on anything available to be put between the teeth. When surgeons "surge," they may "crack" a chest in order to get it open. Notice the power of the (often male) physician which many of these expressions convey.

. . .

The third language can be used to obscure information rather than communicate it. Announcing a "Code 99," or a "Code Blue," or a "Dr. C. Arrest," supposedly avoids unduly alarming other patients and visitors while alerting the hospital staff to an emergency. However, I doubt if many people are fooled by this ploy. Saying that there's a "Code Brown" *is* more esthetic than telling the nurse that a patient's bowel movement needs to be cleaned up.

Physicians might speak to each other of "anaplastic changes" when they don't want to say "cancer" or "tumor" in front of the patient. Or they may use the term "thought disorder" as a euphemism for "schizophrenia." In these cases it's the *manner* in which the words are used rather than the words themselves which make them third language.

. . .

Many medical students see the illnesses of psychiatric patients as "supratentorial" (a pejorative way of saying it's emotional or "in the head"). You might offer such patients "upper deltoid therapy" (patting the patient's shoulder.) Or they may have "hypothorazinemia," meaning that they're on too low of a dose of Thorazine for being so severely mentally ill. A similar term would be "vitamin H deficiency," meaning that the patient could benefit from Haldol. (Both Haldol and Thorazine are registered trademarks for antipsychotic medications.)

Some psychiatric patients are merely "warehoused" (given little active treatment), during which time they are only "fed and watered" (basic needs attended to at appropriate intervals). Perhaps even worse therapeutically is to let them recycle through a "revolving door" every few months. An alternative would be to "turf" patients (transfer elsewhere) by providing "Greyhound Therapy" (assisting with transportation which will allow them to be "dumped" in another town). Prior to a transfer to another ward or hospital, the patient's chart might need to be "buffed" (notes written so that the patients look healthier or more desirable than might actually be the case). As in any specialty, if the patient dies, he or she "buys the farm."

. . .

I'm sure it's obvious by now that doctors frequently speak over the heads of most patients. Some of the third language may seem mildly (or blackly) humorous, such as calling a urologist a "pecker checker." Unfortunately, such terms can also promote an unprofessional atmosphere. Patients who inadvertently hear certain third language terms—and the staff's accompanying joviality—might properly feel demeaned. Would you like to hear your neurologist say he was going to "tend his garden," that is, attend to patients who were comatose ("vegetables").

The third language also leads to misunderstandings. To use the previous example, "tending gardens" has nothing to do with "cabbages." This is the verbal pronunciation of "CABGS" which stands for "coronary artery bypass graft surgery," or "bypass surgery" for short. I recently heard a physician throw out the term "cabbages" on a radio talk show without a second's pause of concern that anyone understood him. The alert host properly asked for a definition. The point here is that physicians simply take our language for granted when we really should know better.

Whatever words caregivers use must be spoken with clarity, compassion, kindness, humanity, consideration, and grace. They need to be *professional* in the manner words are used as well as in their selection.

To the extent that this third language is useful and appropriate, it should be encouraged. It adds a certain color and excitement to ordinary language as it communicates important concepts to students and colleagues.

But, to the extent that it is pejorative and reflects thinking which is unprofessional and prejudicial, it should be eliminated. It helps not a with for students to hear of patients who are "crocks," "gomers," "gorks," and the aforementioned "vegetables"—all negative terms for certain types of patients. The underlying significance of such usage is disturbing. Do they reflect how the speakers actually perceive the patients?

. . .

Of what value is all this to you? This hidden language is certainly eye-opening. More important, knowing that it exists may provide an understanding of some of the attitudes of "professionals" who work with you.

If you want something really practical from the third language, remember this term: "doctors' time." It refers to the 15, 30, or 60 minutes that physicians seem to run behind the rest of the world. Next time you're cooling your heels in a waiting room, you'll at least understand why the doctor doesn't seem much concerned: on "doctor's time," he or she may actually be *ahead* of schedule.

But the most important thing to learn from this chapter is to *ask* when you don't understand what your caregiver is saying. Don't be so awed by the image or presence of a physician that you're reluctant to ask for an explanation of information which may be literally vital to you.

CHAPTER 8

Understanding Treatment and Its Limitations: Surgery—Medical Treatment—Psychotherapy

Pearl:

Ideally, treatment is a frank and interactive effort between patients and caregivers.

The first rule of medicine is "Do no harm." This is an important admonition for all caregivers because of the tremendous potential for today's treatments to both cure and kill.

The duty to avoid harm is usually seen as the responsibility of professionals. But responsibility should be shared by patients and practitioners alike. I don't say this to relieve the burden of the professionals; they still have the major responsibility. Ultimately, however, patients must accept the final responsibility for their own care.

Such sharing is a necessity. First, the modern medical world has demonstrated time and again its failure to live up to its obligation as guardian of the patient. Second, regardless of how vigilant physicians may be, patients can still make very positive contributions not only to their own safety, but to the greater effectiveness of their care as well.

How does sharing work? The physician has the responsibility to adequately inform the patient of treatment options. The patient then has the authority to accept or decline based on an understanding of the treatment's chances of success or failure. And, when people appropriately feel that refusal is the best course, they should decline. The key word, of course, is "appropriately."

Patients can err at both extremes of the decision-making process regarding treatment. At one end ("no"), they sometimes refuse proper care which they perceive as too dangerous. But these patients may be declining appropriate surgeries, medications, or procedures which would actually help them. They need to realize that more serious problems may warrant greater risks.

More likely, patients err at the other end ("yes") by passively agreeing to almost anything their doctor recommends. This is where sharing fails. To make matters worse, history shows that all too often there's not even an illness present in the first place. The consequences of treating non-problems definitely introduces unnecessary risks. Patients with normal tonsils, undergoing the routine delivery of a newborn, or experiencing appropriate sadness may be treated inappropriately as "sick."

Other patients will demand treatment when none is indicated and so must accept at least a minor part of the risk if the physician capitulates, say by agreeing to a Cesarean-section or by prescribing an antibiotic in cases where these aren't indicated.

Physicians are inclined to err on the side of "phys-ishing." That is, when faced with a suffering patient, doctors usually do what they've been trained to do—something, *anything*—run more tests, operate, anything that is active. Giving the patient a prescription is perhaps the most common action. Practitioners feel that the patient has an expectation of getting something and so naturally strive to meet that expectation.

Of surgery I've heard it said that "a chance to cut is a chance to cure." It shouldn't be surprising that if we train someone to do surgery—without including an overall "human perspective" in their education—that they will sometimes "surge" inappropriately when given an opportunity.

So, the patient has a dilemma. He or she is suffering and wants relief. Relief—even for relatively minor problems—can have risks ranging all the way from mild sedation or a little nausea, to major disability or death. The patient should always be aware of this and be prepared to judge his or her treatment's appropriateness. The patient must ultimately decide on risks versus benefits.

To help in these decisions, this chapter will offer some additional comments on treatment, including some general guidelines for patients. Then surgery, medication, and psychotherapy (the most common treatments) will be discussed individually. Finally, I'll present an approach for evaluating progress once treatment has started.

. . .

In discussing treatment, an important sequence for success can be easily overlooked: Proper treatment generally follows an accurate diagnosis—a fact which can't be emphasized too strongly. Except by occasional sheer coincidence and luck, all the expensive care in the world won't help when applied to the wrong condition. Making an incorrect diagnosis is both easier and more frequent than many patients suspect. So important is this topic that misdiagnoses and "undiagnosable" conditions will be considered in a separate chapter.

Physicians often are uncertain of a diagnosis. However, they are astute enough to realize that frequently an exact diagnosis (and subsequent "proper treatment") doesn't make much difference in the long run. Most visits to doctors aren't matters of life or death. Most patients will eventually get better anyway and suffer no serious adverse effects from a prescribed course of treatment based on an incorrect diagnosis. Physicians are fortunate that they are able to get so many people in for office appointments before they get better on their own. Even in health care, "timing is everything." Physicians do try very hard to avoid missing those diagnoses which are both serious and treatable—and for which prompt attention is important.

If there is reasonable continuity of care—along with a satisfactory patient-doctor relationship—the physician can probably count on the patient returning if the problem persists or worsens or new symptoms appear. At that point, the diagnosis may be clearer, more testing can be done, or treatment can be altered. A more on-target treatment can then be given at this later time, usually without any significant complications from the delay. This is part of the reason that managed care—as bad as it can be at times—can continue to look fairly good from the perspective of outcome. And since managed care will usually provide as little attention as possible—correct or incorrect—it actually can play a role in preventing unnecessary complications by reducing the amount of unnecessary treatment.

The very best approach to treatment is to not require any. That is to say that *prevention* should be everyone's primary goal, even before good treatment. As in aviation, it's better to skillfully avoid problems (such as flying into bad weather) rather than to skillfully deal with them (such as having to survive flying out of that weather).

Treatment has financial consequences as well as significant clinical ramifications. Look, for example, at people who visit doctors because of common complaints, such as headaches, backaches, respiratory trouble, or GI symptoms. I'd say that only about 50 percent of the time is there likely to be enough physical benefit incurred to have made these visits worthwhile. (This ballpark figure is simply my educated guess.) Regardless, the visits cost plenty and entail risks.

This isn't to say that a person with these complaints shouldn't see a physician. Often a cure isn't possible (such as with a cold or a terminal illness), but physical and emotional *relief* from symptoms may be. Simply seeing a doctor often lessens worry and provides reassurance for many people.

But there's a price to pay for reassurance, anything from side effects from medications (which range from inconvenient to life-threatening), to complications from recommended procedures. Even relatively simple diagnostic procedures can be dangerous: A newspaper reported the death of a patient allegedly as the result of positioning the head for a CAT scan. Complications are in addition to the time and financial cost to the patient. You, as a patient, must be prepared to say *stop*.

Many factors go into the selection of a treatment program by a physician. More and more, physicians are working from published guidelines for treating specific problems. "If the patient has this, then you do that." This is a relatively new development in medicine, and its overall success has yet to be adequately assessed. It certainly gives concern that the future lies more in "cookbook" medicine than in individualized attention. It also allows—for better or for worse—application of complex approaches by less well-trained providers who simply follow the book.

However, the treatment process is hardly as cut and dried as "I'll recommend whatever the scientific evidence says to do." To start with, the scientific evidence often is not clear. There may be many acceptable approaches to the same problem. Either surgery or medication can sometimes be legitimate options for a single ailment. And if medications are used, the practitioner can be faced with a bewildering number of choices.

Non-scientific issues also enter into—and may even become the deciding factors—in the selection of treatment. A host of these are known to almost every physician: availability of local resources, advertisements targeted at both the physician and (with more and more frequency these days) the patient, insurance coverage, legal concerns, pressure from managed care, the physician's particular biases and training background, the expectations of the patient, and cost-effectiveness; to name a few.

Pharmacists sometimes use a mortar and pestle to contain and mix the ingredients which are blended together into a prescription. I've suggested to medical students to consider the "ingredients" which go into decision-making in much the same way. The factors described in the paragraph above are poured into the mortar in various proportions and stirred by the pestle of the provider's mind. The final product—a huge combination of factors—is expressed as a recommendation to "take this" or "do that." This might not be a bad analogy for patients to keep in mind as well.

. . .

As a patient, what can you do to affect your treatment? Here are some guidelines.

First, it's important to have an appreciation for some of the limitations of modern care, to understand what's feasible and what's not. For instance, no matter how uncomfortable a viral sore throat may be, all the antibiotics in the world won't help. No matter how expert a psychotherapist may be, the psychological wounds of a lifetime can't be instantly remedied.

A practical mindset—and a plan—also helps. The patient might think something like this: "Maybe a doctor's visit will help me; hopefully it won't hurt me; if I don't get the relief I need, then I'll respond with a return visit, an appointment with another physician, and/or my own further research." Or, the patient might be more succinct and concrete: "I'll go. I'll be vigilant. I'll follow the "Four Steps to Better Care."

An important contributor to successful treatment is continuity of care. This implies that the physician and patient work together over a period of time.

A physician may be able to help a person much more when he or she has a general "feel" for the patient and for the manner in which the patient presents symptoms. Additionally, with time, a trust and a bond can be developed which assists both patient and doctor in more successful treatment.

Treatment is often only as good as its monitoring. That is, even the correct approach may need careful observation and adjustment over a series of visits. Sometimes *only* monitoring the patient's condition, without using any medication, is the best treatment.

The value of the visit is often limited by what the patient is able to understand of the doctor's advice. The physician may feel that he or she is offering a clear and concise explanation of diagnosis and treatment. But, taking in new information in a stressful setting isn't easy. A patient who doesn't understand what is being said should ask for clarification. An airline captain guiding a 747 doesn't feel embarrassed to ask the air traffic controller to "say again,"—neither should you. Requesting written instructions and printed material can also go a long way in overcoming a lack of comprehension.

Ultimately, the patient, not the doctor, must make the decision whether or not to accept treatment. It is the patient who must weigh the risks and benefits of the proposed course of action. While the physician's recommendation should be taken quite seriously, the final authority resides with the one whose life will be primarily affected—that's you. If you are not comfortable with the diagnosis and/or treatment recommendations, then it may be time to exercise both responsibility and authority by declining and/or going elsewhere. These are serious steps and should be taken cautiously. They may have ramifications regarding further care or even insurance coverage.

Surgery

Surgery is certainly one of the most dramatic aspects of health care. It is also one which usually instills the most fear in patients. One of the biggest stains upon the surgical profession is the issue of unnecessary surgery. Tonsillectomies, hysterectomies, and C-sections have become some of the most over-done procedures. Such unnecessary surgery results not only in huge expense but, more importantly, it may result in human tragedy.

It's been said that surgeons look at the human body as a sack of potentially removable organs. While this is a somewhat dark view, it should serve as a warning to patients. At a very minimum, patients should get a clear statement from the surgeon as to why they need a procedure, what would the alternatives be, and what would happen if they declined. Are there alternative medication approaches or non-surgical procedures? A good question for patients to ask any doctor is, "What is the most reasonable *conservative* approach to my problem?"

My best advice on surgery? Get a second opinion. Surgery of any magnitude at all is a serious business. I don't think it should be entered into—except in the most urgent or obvious of circumstances—unless another independent opinion (preferably by someone totally unacquainted with the first surgeon) has been obtained. This re-evaluation should provide both a diagnosis of the problem, as well as a discussion of any available treatment options.

For myself, I'd exclude most minor surgeries from my caution to get a second opinion. The problem is, it can be hard to draw a sharp line between what is major and what is minor. Here's a not-infallible rule of thumb: if the procedure requires the services of an anesthetist or anesthesiologist to assist with pain control, it probably should require a second opinion.

People sometimes overlook the fact that they are paying for the surgeon's judgment as much as his or her surgical skill. I want a surgeon who can feel my abdomen and—where appropriate—say, "No, I think it's best to watch this a little longer before any decision to operate." Even better would be a surgeon who could honestly say, "I think we can handle this without operating."

The expression, "There is no substitute for experience," finds some of its most useful application in the field of surgery. If I were going to have an operation, I would want some assurance that its performance was "old hat" to my surgeon (and to the hospital where it would be performed).

It is quite permissible to ask the surgeon how often he or she does a particular procedure. Although you may not have comparative statistics at hand, the surgeon's answer may give you a general notion of experience with that particular procedure. If the reply is, "This will be the first gallbladder I've removed in two years," then obviously, you may want to re-think your options. If the surgeon seems uncomfortable addressing your question, that may also be a warning sign.

Another way of improving one's chances for getting greater expertise is by moving up the specialty or sub-specialty chain. For instance, a family practitioner probably rarely, if ever, does colon surgery: A general surgeon may work on the colon with some frequency. However, a colon and rectal surgeon may be doing such procedures on a daily basis. Even if you get a specialist, find out if the doctor or a resident under supervision will actually do the procedure.

. . .

Like patients themselves, medical students are awed by the power of the surgeon. They see this specialist as the quintessential healer: Get in, get out, and the disease is gone. Students are usually surprised when I tell them that I place surgeons relatively low on the list of those who cure. Just add together all the unnecessary surgery, all the disability and deaths resulting even from needed operations, the surgeries which are done for relief rather than cure, those which are done for cosmetic purposes, and those for which there are non-surgical alternatives. There's not as much curing going on in those operating rooms as may appear at first glance. Perhaps we should more carefully re-evaluate who cures and who doesn't.

Medical Treatment

As compared to surgical treatment, receiving good medical treatment—that is, being treated with medication or other non-surgical approaches—involves a different emphasis. An operation is a process with a set beginning and ending. It's dramatic. Results—for better or for worse—may be apparent almost immediately. But medical treatment may be prolonged, subtle, and slow in showing progress or failure.

The success of medical treatment is largely contingent upon not one, but a number of small steps well taken. These start with proper diagnosis based on an adequate medical history, examination, and sometimes testing. The steps proceed through an explanation of the findings, treatment, and treatment alternatives. Then comes an agreement by the patient and doctor after careful discussion and consideration. Finally, there may be a period of monitoring the progress of the patient on the proposed treatment plan and making adjustments when indicated.

Throughout the course of treatment, attention to detail remains vitally important. Doctors usually keep written records of the patient's progress. But for the patient, keeping a personal clinical diary can also be a very effective tool. This can be used to keep track of symptoms and treatment results as well as possible adverse reactions to any medication. Such information can then be shared with the treating physician or passed on to subsequent doctors. Additionally, the patient should use the time during the illness for further reading in order to understand his problem more thoroughly.

As far as possible, medication should be taken when, and as, directed. But, since there are often alternative dosing strategies available, inquire about these. Pharmacists can be good additional sources for this kind of information. Sometimes a medication being taken three times a day can be taken just as effectively on a once-a-day schedule. But talk with your doctor before actually making any changes in medication scheduling.

Physicians usually proceed with medical treatment using the concept of "horses and zebras." Just as the sound of hoof beats coming down a road would likely be more commonly associated with horses (rather than zebras) in this country, particular symptoms are closely associated with particular common diagnoses. For example, a backache is probably more often due to a strain, sprain, or arthritis (horse) rather than a slipped disc (zebra). Likewise, a headache is more likely due to tension than to a brain tumor.

Especially in a managed care setting where there may be a greater emphasis on cost-effectiveness, the physician is far more likely to initially choose a "horse" to fit the symptom even though the final diagnosis may ultimately turn out to be a "zebra." There is *usually* nothing intrinsically wrong with this approach, as long as the patient is being monitored carefully. It assumes that the consequences of harm in the meantime are likely to be slim because of any delay in alternate treatment. It also assumes that any critical condition which required immediate attention has been ruled out.

. . .

There are a number of additional aspects of medical care which I will mention briefly. Although the first rule of medicine is "do no harm," physicians have been known to develop something of an immunity to concern over the side effects of their medications and other treatments. The physician knows that serious medication complications occur in only a very small percentage of patients. However, if you are that patient, then it happens 100 percent to you. So be sure that the most significant side effects are explained to you so that you may consider them beforehand and are willing to accept the risk(s).

Another point: People should get the medications they need in adequate dosages. However, I often see abuses in this area when too many medications are used at dosages that are too high. This is especially unfortunate if only minor symptoms are being treated, or if complications caused by the inappropriate use of other medications are the problem. Work out a program with your physician that will provide as many medications as are necessary, but no more. They should be prescribed at as high of a dose as you need, but no higher. Be involved in the selection of a medication program. Ask questions. Know the alternatives. Be sure you get answers.

It's primarily the physician's responsibility to ask the patient about medications he or she may already be taking. However, if an additional drug is being considered, the patient may have to take the initiative to remind the doctor of other medications he or she is taking. This can help to avoid unfortunate—even fatal—drug interactions. As patients are prescribed more and more medications, the possibility of drug interactions become more of a problem.

Finally, just because you get better after starting a medication don't assume that there's a direct "cause-and-effect" relationship. Medicines can have strong placebo effects. Both patient and doctor should be aware of this in evaluating the response to a program of treatment. This knowledge can help you avoid taking (and paying for) basically ineffective drugs. Additionally, sometimes people seem to improve on medication even though they would have gotten better without any help at all. The body often has marvelous self-curative powers. After all, throughout history, most people have gotten over most of their illnesses most of the time; otherwise, none of us would be here alive today.

. . .

Psychotherapy

It has been said, tongue-in-cheek, that anyone who goes to see a psychiatrist should have his or her head examined. I fully agree with that warning, assuming it means that there should be a thorough evaluation prior to any recommendation for psychotherapy or medications. Unfortunately, even having an evaluation by a psychiatrist is no guarantee that physical causes will be recognized.

It's no wonder that psychotherapy is obscure to most lay people: I've heard the total number of different kinds of psychotherapy (such as Freudian, Jungian, and cognitive behavioral) put into the hundreds. While this may be an exaggeration, the fact is that any list of all the various "schools" would be quite lengthy.

There is also a variety of therapists to choose from including psychiatrists (M.D.'s), psychologists, social workers, and others. And an individual therapist—a psychiatrist for instance—may offer treatment approaches from a number of different schools.

Incompetent psychotherapy can be just as harmful to a person's life as incompetent surgery. The downside of poor therapy is not only a continuation or worsening of the distress, but—depending on the illness—there can be a serious risk of suicide or even danger to others. The illness can also have tremendous effects on the quality of life of family and friends. And, of course, the "prescription of self" by the therapist (patient - therapist sex) is always inappropriate in my opinion.

One type of psychotherapy many people know of is psychoanalysis, probably the most expensive and prolonged form of therapy. This is not a negative comment about psychoanalysis. When used appropriately, it is a marvelous treatment. In addition to being a form of therapy, psychoanalysis is also a psychology which underlies much of modern mental health care. Some incorrectly equate psychoanalysis with just about any form of psychotherapy, assuming that anyone in therapy is in "analysis." Psychoanalysis is actually relatively rare these days. It requires an *extremely* lengthy training period. A major reason for its decline is that it's simply too expensive for many patients to afford.

Therapy doesn't have to be prolonged in all cases. Sometimes even a single visit can be productive. More typically, the number of sessions may run from perhaps 5 to 25. The cost can be anywhere from no fee at a community mental health center, to $100 or more an hour at a private office. (By comparison, one of my attorneys charges $235 an hour.)

Psychotherapy represents a unique relationship between patient and therapist in which both cooperate to resolve the distress by means of utilizing the minds of both. This statement may be as close as I can come to actually defining psychotherapy (no small task!). Of course, there are variations on this theme, including therapy groups.

It may well be that all the various psychotherapies are more similar than they are different. Dr. Jerome Frank has insightfully written that the various therapies share common characteristics such as (1) relationship, (2) rationale, and (3) ritual. That is, they all involve a unique bond of patient and therapist, operate from some particular theoretical framework, and involve a specific activity or activities. Because of these shared healing characteristics, one may work just as well as another for a given patient. But for some problems, specific kinds of therapy are indicated.

Psychotherapy, when well done, can literally be a godsend for the patient. Even on a purely philosophical basis, it's a beautiful concept where two people work earnestly together to benefit the one in distress. Such an approach should provide a confidential setting in which material can be dealt with non-judgmentally. I consider confidentiality and being non-judgmental to be the two keystones of the patient-therapist relationship. Neither may be easy to preserve in a managed care environment.

Good practitioners of psychotherapy require as much expertise as do good surgeons. It may seem like just "talking," but much skill and understanding are involved. "Listening" is so important in this activity that it might even be better called "listening therapy."

My medical students often want to know, "Who are the best therapists?" I tell them that the best therapists are those who are the best therapists. By that, I mean that academic degrees, while valuable indicators of a certain level of attainment, are not as important as the personal characteristics of the individual therapist. These include professionalism, empathy, and interpersonal skills. I am sure that there are many nurses and social workers who are far better therapists than some psychologists and psychiatrists.

In *general*, I think psychiatrists usually don't make very good therapists, for several reasons. They are often very busy and subsequently don't have the time to provide regularly scheduled psychotherapy appointments as might be indicated. Many don't give credence to psychotherapy; they're more likely to see a problem as "biological" than are most other mental health workers. Psychiatrists often spend such a large amount of time focused on learning and practicing medication management that little time is available to develop expertise in psychotherapy. On a practical level, psychiatrists doing psychotherapy fit in poorly with today's managed care philosophy. A third-party payer is unlikely to reimburse them at $100 an hour for something a social worker may be willing and/or competent to do for half the price.

If I had to blindly pick someone to help me without knowing anything else about the therapist, I would probably select a psychologist. It has been my general impression that, overall, psychologists offer the best combination of training, availability, and affability.

Picking a therapist shouldn't be confused with choosing someone to do an evaluation of a problem. In theory, at least, psychiatrists should be the best qualified to most comprehensively look at the *cause* of the distress. As M.D.'s, they've been trained both biologically and psychologically. In practice, not all psychiatrists do a very good job of evaluation since their search for a cause may be heavily skewed by a biological bias. So their recommendations may lean toward a "quick fix" with medication even when psychotherapy is indicated.

There is an ethical issue involving diagnosis which I'm asked about again and again when I speak to mental health professionals. They recognize that insurers will only pay for therapy regarding specific diagnoses. They ask if they should falsify records in order to obtain coverage. What they decide will determine whether *your* diagnosis will be based on fact or fiction. Find out in advance how your insurance works.

How do you find a good therapist? It can be difficult to get recommendations from other patients because of the stigma attached to being in treatment. You may have to depend more heavily on your physician for recommendations than upon friends and relatives.

You may have to meet with more than one therapist prior to commencing treatment with anyone. While the therapist is interviewing you, there's nothing wrong with you interviewing the therapist. Hopefully, one of these visits will bring you into contact with an individual who you consider to be open, professional, and with whom you have a reasonable level of comfort. Ask potential candidates to discuss with you both their treatment philosophy, as well as the practical aspects of their treatment (fees, office hours, availability, what a treatment session actually consists of). Ask them how they "see" your problem at least in a general way and how they would approach its treatment. If they don't give answers with which you are comfortable, consider seeing someone else. But use your common sense as much as possible: Don't necessarily eliminate a possible therapist just on the basis of seeing things differently. The therapist may well be correct.

Psychotherapy is a relationship in which it is especially important for you to rely on your own judgment and impressions of the practitioner. Your "gut feelings" may ultimately be the best source of information available to you. Of course, your choice may be limited by supply, distance, fees, or type of insurance coverage.

A confounding factor is the question of the use of medication along with psychotherapy. This is an extremely complex issue. On the surface, at least, these two approaches would seem to be diametrically opposed to each other. (Why take drugs if the problem is psychological? Why have psychotherapy if the problem is biological?) That is not necessarily the case. At a minimum, you can ask the therapist to explain the rationale for the use of both approaches simultaneously if such a plan is recommended to you.

. . .

One final note on psychotherapy: Sometimes we overvalue its potential. Many people come to therapy not because they are "mentally ill" but because they are simply unhappy about their situation in life or their lack of progression towards goals. They may be bored with routine or discouraged by the realities of life.

Therapy may be of assistance in these cases, but it shouldn't be seen as the *only* possible solution. Depending upon the circumstances, any of the following might be better solutions: a personal self-evaluation of one's life, a change to a more satisfying career, a vacation, walks in the woods or mountains, reading great literature, talking with family or friends, taking a look at the role of religion in one's life, or a philosophical consideration of the meaning of that life.

I think we need to be cautious even of what we *call* psychotherapy. For example, I offer "personal consulting" to "clients" (not patients), an activity which I don't believe meets the criteria for "therapy." Basically, I function as an educational resource for those who simply wish to discuss distressing, but non-clinical issues with a knowledgeable individual. In essence, I'm a "smart, paid friend." This is only for people who elect not to work within a formal mental health setting and who don't appear to require such a setting.

Additional information with regard to mental illness (including medication approaches) in contained in Chapter Thirteen.

. . .

Successful treatment of any type is the culmination of a lengthy and complex process which begins with adequate access to the system and continues through proper evaluation, a discussion of any appropriate treatments or alternatives, and ongoing management, if required. Throughout, the process must be customed-tailored to the patient as carefully as any fine suit of clothes.

Many times the best treatment is no treatment at all. Physicians use a number of phrases which allude to this: "time is the best healer," "tincture of time," "benign neglect," and even "masterful neglect." It may be the task of the patient to secure the best non-treatment available. No student of mine leaves training without learning that—in the appropriate circumstance—it's quite permissible to do nothing (except to provide comfort to the patient).

Regardless of the exact type of treatment, be wary of agreeing to work with anyone who is being supervised. This could range from a nursing student to a senior resident physician. I'm not saying don't work with them, but at least be both selective and extra cautious. After all, there's a reason they are getting supervision. Be sure you understand in advance the division of labor between your doctor and any trainees under his or her direction. This is especially important with regard to surgery.

. . .

How can patients tell if their treatment is satisfactory? Unfortunately, there is no sure-fire formula. But, the following questions—when considered together—may help you in this important determination:

1. At a common-sense level, do you feel comfortable that the diagnosis is correct? Have there been tests or X-rays to confirm the diagnosis, when appropriate? Does the physician's explanation of the treatment plans make sense to you based on the diagnosis? Does it all fit with what you've read and researched? If there are inconsistencies, what are the results of your efforts to resolve them?

2. Is your recovery (or relief) following a course you would have expected based on your own study or upon your doctor's prediction? Are you "on schedule?"

3. Is there objective clinical evidence of improvement (e.g., changes in blood tests or on X-rays)?

4. Is there objective evidence of improvement in your life? (Fewer hospitalizations? More mobility? An

improvement in weight or a normalization of sleep hours? More workdays?)

5. Has a consultation ("second opinion") been obtained because of the seriousness or complications of your ailment, or its slow progress? What does the consultant say? What does your own physician say of your progress? Does he or she seem more or less at ease and open in discussions during visits?

6. Is the treatment program being simplified over time—fewer medications, lower dosage, fewer office visits, less testing, and so on?

7. Do you feel you've been kept well-informed, especially if there has been slow progress?

8. Has there been one or more unexpected complications or untoward events? How has your physician responded to these?

9. Has there been an air of timeliness to your care? Do delays seem excessive for tests, consultations, return visits with your doctor? In the hospital, does the staff respond with reasonable promptness and attend adequately to your needs?

10. And finally, are you enjoying life more and "suffering" less—are you simply "feeling better?"

Use these ten points as an overall evaluation of your care. But every point may not apply in every case; they must be taken in proper context. Your physician may have to help you evaluate some of them. If these questions bring troubling answers consider such alternatives as trying to resolve the issue with your physician, getting a consultation (or *another* consultation), switching doctors, doing more personal research, and so on.

. . .

Be reasonable in your expectations of treatment. Carefully weigh the risks and benefits. Monitor your own care using the ten points given above. You are the one who will pay the real price if treatment fails, not the doctors or other caregivers.

Occasionally, reality must take precedence over expectations. Sometimes all a physician can offer is a willingness to share in the patient's suffering while he or she endures that for which there is no other answer.

CHAPTER 9

Understanding the "Biz-Med Complex"

Pearl:

Failure to understand the Biz-Med Complex limits our potential for better care.

Legend has it that Alexander the Great needed just one blow of his sword to sever the Gordian Knot which had defied all efforts to untie it. Our health care system is modern society's Gordian Knot. But, where is our Alexander and his sword?

Referring to our nation's overall approach to health care as a system may be giving it more credit than is due. What we have is more like a rudderless ship floundering on a turbulent sea. The "S.S. Health Care Chaos" might be a more appropriate metaphor.

And it is an absolutely enormous ship. A phenomenal number of people in a multitude of different professions and businesses are directly involved. Each incredibly complex part of the vessel has an equally complex relationship with all the other parts, and the complexity feeds upon itself as these parts interact.

It's not surprising that outsiders (patients) get discouraged and frustrated in trying to understand this system as it impacts upon their personal health care—as well as upon the nation's health care. Insiders (providers) get discouraged and frustrated as well! While everyone would like to "put it all together," the task simply seems overwhelming. Patients jump ship first, assuming the system is beyond their comprehension, and simply turn the steering over to the pros. The pros, however, are also puzzled, and so the ship remains adrift.

. . .

High on anyone's list of significant people and facilities involved in health care would be some of those already discussed in detail: doctors, hospitals, and nurses. The basic duties of these three groups are defined simply enough, but the scope of these duties is huge. Physicians must practice medicine, nurses must provide care at the bedside and in other settings, hospitals must provide extremely sophisticated services for the seriously ill.

But, physicians also teach medical students, fight encroachment into their territory, and concern themselves with the administrative aspect of their practice—in addition to numerous other activities. Nurses search for their professional identity, work to expand their roles, and deal with the psychological burdens of their careers. Hospitals must not only provide an environment for quality care, but they must stay financially solvent and satisfy their governing bodies while doing so.

The list of organizations and professionals, their myriad duties, and how they should be helping you goes on and on. Often, the boundaries separating one from the other are unclear to patients and professionals alike.

How involved is this system? The following is an incomplete list of what makes up the Biz-Med Complex, but it certainly points up why patients often feel confused and powerless.

Physicians
Hospitals
Nurses

Clinics
Professional Organizations (e.g., the AMA)
Technicians (X-ray, laboratory, etcetera)
Dentists
Podiatrists
Physical Therapists
Recreational Therapists
Social Workers
Psychologists
Hospital Administrators
Managed Care/Fee-For-Service Firms
Lawyers Practicing in Health Care Areas
Manufacturers of Durable Goods (e.g., hospital beds, technical and surgical equipment)
Manufactures of Disposable Medical Supplies
Distributors of Disposable Medical Supplies and Durable Goods
Architects of Medical Facilities
Medical Schools
Nursing Schools
Health-Related Government Agencies
Medical Textbooks (Writers, Publishers, Bookstores)
Medical Waste Disposal
Ethicists
Pharmaceutical Companies
Drugstores and Pharmacists
Ambulance Services & Ambulance Staffs
Home Health Care Services
Nursing Homes
Accreditation & Certification Organizations
Physician Assistants
Researchers & Research Facilities
Businesses Involved in Medical Conventions & Seminars
Administrative Consultants
Marketers for Medical Services & Supplies

Various Charities
Board Members of Firms/Organizations on This List
Shareholders in Firms on This List

. . .

The "Biz-Med Complex" is a designation (introduced in Chapter One) which I use to include all the people, organizations, and businesses involved in delivering health care. This term also gives a suggestion of the financial aspects of the medical world. The fact that I tie money and health care together in this way is not a negative comment: It is realistic. In fact, in some elements of the Complex, such as charities, money is a means to largely altruistic ends. My concern is the extent to which money becomes the focal point. Operationally, the Biz-Med Complex is driven by the same thing that strongly drives the patient-doctor relationship—patient vulnerability. This vulnerability, in turn, drives the finances.

Now, my list is surely not given to imply that all those who are included are money-hungry scavengers feeding upon the ill. Most have the patient's best interest at heart. And, many of these organizations and businesses are ethically and efficiently run. This list is simply given as a starting point to show the extent of the Biz-Med Complex. Progressing to an understanding of the Complex will take some additional effort.

The real question here is whether or not the Biz-Med Complex serves us well. It is a delicately balanced system, intimately interdependent. Everything within it is connected to—but not necessarily *integrated* with—every other part. And the entire Biz-Med Complex is connected to the larger society. Anyone attempting to improve health care by making changes within parts of the Complex should first understand health care and the consequences of altering its delivery. Changes can result in far-reaching effects both inside and outside of the Biz-Med Complex.

The bigger something is, the more momentum it has. Our behemoth of a health care system will keep rumbling along unless significant force is brought to change its direction. "Significant" doesn't necessarily mean "dramatic" (as in gigantic government programs), although it might.

. . .

The size and chaos of the Biz-Med Complex calls out for some sort of organizing principles. What threads do—or should—run through its organizations and groups to enable them to fulfill their critical tasks? And what understanding can we come to regarding them?

Primary among these threads would be professionalism, which requires high standards of excellence, education or training, honesty, ethics, and performance. If there was true professionalism throughout the entire Biz-Med Complex, one could make a reasonable argument that no reform or other superimposed constraints would be necessary.

Another organizing thread would be an adequate educational system which is geared to providing a sufficient number of qualified caregivers and other workers within the Complex. These people would be taught to give more than lip service to the concept of the "whole person." Health care professionals would be trained to treat *people who are suffering*, not to simply treat diseases.

Much of the schooling of health care professionals in this country is funded by taxpayers. Therefore, it would be perfectly acceptable for us to expect these schools to provide adequate numbers of caregivers. In spite of cries from medical schools that larger classes would dilute the number of qualified applicants, there is a huge pool of capable and very "human" people who would jump at the opportunity for consideration. Many would make excellent physicians. Or, perhaps we could consider those nurses who want expanded roles in health care. I think much enthusiasm is likely to be found among nurses for acquiring an M.D. degree if this could be accomplished efficiently.

Effective, but limited, government involvement could provide a third major thread in this whole fabric. This could include financial support for those patients falling "between the cracks;" research where the tremendous resources of the government might appropriately be called upon (e.g., AIDS); having less waste in that part of the federal bureaucracy already dealing with health care; and public health efforts such as immunizations, assisting in mass disasters, and tracking epidemics. (We'll talk more about government involvement in Chapter 25.) Perhaps most importantly, dedicated government leaders could provide some of the missing moral leadership to help reverse the chaos with which we are now involved.

. . .

There is one stronger thread which could be used to bundle together the previous mentioned threads. That would be *recognition of a joint mission* by all those involved in the Biz-Med Complex.

All or most of the organizations and groups mentioned in the earlier list are likely to have their own mission statements (some should be taken with a grain of salt as they often represent public relations platitudes). But the Biz-Med Complex doesn't have an agreed upon, mutually acceptable, overriding statement which could provide vision for, and leadership to, the whole. To develop such a statement would take a great deal of coordination and effort. But imagine if everyone in the Complex worked under the following premise:

> "Those of us whose work involves health care services, products, and related needs, will strive cooperatively to provide every American with access to quality products and services, working as partners with citizens, which is in *everyone's* best interest."

The government might have to remove some of its restrictive regulatory stances (for instance, involving mergers) to allow a mission statement like this to be implemented. But, considering some of the proposals which have recently been put forth for changes in health care, this step wouldn't be all that drastic, especially when you take into account the possible benefits.

Even though I am not a fan of government bureaucracy, perhaps we should push for the creation of one new agency which could spearhead the push for an overriding mission statement: "The Office of What's Really Wrong with Health Care & How the Government Can Provide Leadership so that the Rest of Us Can Correct It."

. . .

It's worthwhile to point out that weaving together the above-mentioned threads will still not create an ideal system. Some imperfect patients will always be attended by some imperfect caregivers. And, unless there's massive (and unwanted) government takeover of the entire Biz-Med Complex, enterprises involved in health care will need to continue to operate with a keen eye toward profits.

As I indicated earlier, there is nothing wrong with making money. People often complain about pharmaceutical companies and the insurance industry, which have to make money to survive, forgetting that such organizations are not charities. They are willing to provide us with what we pay them for, be it a medication or an insurance contract. We sometimes unfairly castigate them when they resist going beyond providing a quality product or meeting the terms of their agreements.

Perhaps, adhering to the mission statement given above, these firms could be more informative regarding not only what they do offer, but what they don't. Consumers would then have a better understanding of what they can expect. And providers and consumers could work more cooperatively with each other.

. . .

There's a fact that most ordinary people recognize, even if those within the Biz-Med Complex always do not: Health care delivery is not only complex, but flawed. No amount of government intervention or internal changes can make this go away. But even given its complexity and problems, most Americans *could* understand and participate meaningfully in health care delivery. Currently though, how many of us even bother to read our insurance policies with the same care that we read the owner's manual for our new automobiles?

Chaos can and should be minimized. This could be accomplished, in part, by bringing together the organizing threads for the Biz-Med Complex mentioned earlier, especially the development of a comprehensive mission statement.

Improvement originating from within is only one option for our nation's health care. Of course, care could just remain unchanged—and some would argue that wouldn't be such a bad idea. Care could also be turned upside down by government fiat. Or, the government could encourage less drastic alterations. Finally, some combination of the above could occur. Obviously, there are many possibilities. Whoever might try to implement change within the Complex had better know what they're doing.

If all else fails—or perhaps along with other efforts—we may have to become our own personal Alexander (or Alexandra) the Great in an effort to undo the Gordian Knot of our own personal health care.

PART 2

Getting Better Care

CHAPTER 10

The Doctors Appointment

Pearl:
The patient can influence the value of an appointment even more than the doctor.

The very complex interaction between patient and doctor during an appointment can be likened to theater. It is well-rehearsed, well-orchestrated, and just about everyone knows what's going on behind the scenes—except the patients, who are paying the price of admission. While sometimes reduced to a comedy of errors, this visit ideally resembles a drama with a satisfying ending.

As in the theater, everyone has his or her assigned role to play. In "traditional medical theater," the doctor is the hero, the patient is the protagonist, and suffering is the villain. There is a potentially large supporting cast including the office staff and, occasionally, family members of the patient.

Between the lead performers—the doctor and the patient—there should be a chemistry. These two play off each other, constantly parrying and thrusting. A variety of deeply felt emotions come naturally: arrogance, fear, anxiety, hope, anger, desperation, suffering, relief, and even joy and happiness.

Behind the scenes is meticulous preparation, long rehearsals (especially by the doctor), and an impressive array of clinical props. Above all, there is the script and its well-defined roles. The doctor knows the script almost to perfection. The patient, however, has stumbled upon an unfamiliar scene. He is like an ill-prepared stand-in suddenly thrust onto center stage. Will the patient succeed? Can he be a star?

While the villain (suffering) is the major problem, close behind are the complications which arise when the players—especially the patient and the doctor—fail to follow the script or step out of character. This drama, as usually enacted in modern life, requires adherence to the lines. This is not improvisational theater: To ad-lib is to disrupt the smooth flow of the action. If not properly handled, unexpected changes can irritate the doctor, further confuse the patient, and even jeopardize care.

The doctor is a wise, all-knowing, parent-figure to be obeyed. The patient is a mildly interesting character, but ignorant and an object of pity. If the patient gets swept up with the flow of the action and follows the doctor's lead, the plot can move quickly—but perhaps imperfectly—to completion.

Unfortunately, characters view the action differently. Success for the patient may be survival and the relief of his suffering. Success for the doctor may be accurate diagnosis, cutting-edge treatment, a fee, and perhaps some ego massage. Success for the office staff may be a paycheck and a pat on the head by the doctor for stellar performances in their supporting roles.

. . .

Part One, "Looking Behind the Sterile Curtain," gave you some insight into the training and the psyche of physicians. You saw their strengths: hard-working, bright, extensively trained, and usually well-meaning and competent. You also learned their weaknesses: socially isolated and intellectually narrow, harmed as well as benefited by their training, and often discouraged and controlling. At their best they are caring, dedicated, and professional; at their worst, they are greedy, dishonest, and arrogant.

Now it's time to see how the characteristics of the physician influence what happens in an outpatient setting: The doctor's office. More importantly, you'll discover options for responding to the problems when they arise.

Before we begin, however, the "Four Steps to Better Care" bear repeating for this setting. A more successful office visit can result from *understanding* what is happening during the visit (the *process*). This knowledge is a remedy for what otherwise might appear chaotic, too complex, and even overwhelming. Your active *involvement* can counteract being intentionally or unintentionally excluded from the decision-making process. Taking *responsibility* for your own health is a protection from caregivers who would be less than thorough, professional, or responsible. And, after you are fully informed, you should exercise your *authority* to accept or decline the recommendations of others—or even to take the initiative of making your own suggestions.

The office is the setting for a very complex interaction of patient and doctor. Neither participant is fully aware of all the interactions as the encounter proceeds. I hope this section will make some of the underlying dynamics more evident for you. It will also help you to see why much of what occurs between patient and doctor is beyond the reach of legislation or of being "managed" from the outside.

You've already seen that doctors are no more or less human than their patients. Their training and work is different than yours, but their degrees don't put them above you.

So at the start of any encounter, in your own mind, you can strip away the doctor's inhibiting facade so that you can stand before each other on equal psychological footing to accomplish your common task. Without unnecessary barriers (for example, the doctor's almost god-like aura) standing between the two of you, your mutual effort can be more productive.

And remember: Probably no one is better equipped to be in charge of your care than you are. While doctors will usually put your best interests first, they cannot always be depended upon to look beyond their own pressures and needs. They and the medical world will too often focus upon themselves—not you. Even when they act in what they perceive as the most helpful fashion to the patient, their perceptions—largely formed during training—are not always accurate.

. . .

No two clinical cases are ever alike. The combination of you and your illness at a particular point in time is a unique situation. If you wish for it to be attended to in a manner befitting that uniqueness, then you must arrange it. This is not just the doctor's responsibility.

You should work to forge a therapeutic partnership with the doctor. He should be the *junior* partner and you the senior. In the lingo of the business world, "He will report to you." Here is the best "job description" I can give you in your role as an outpatient:

> Know that you have the responsibility to talk meaningfully with your physician whether or not he is comfortable with that approach. Insist that he hears and understands you, responds to your questions and needs, makes his diagnosis and treatment clear to you, explains the options and addresses your concerns. Insist that you be allowed to get involved. Understand both the process of health care and the health care problem itself—and monitor both carefully. Know that you have the final authority. But do all this in the most open, pleasant, and receptive fashion of which you are capable. Do it

after careful preparation and within an appropriate context.

Can you have any faith in your physician? Of course—but it must be *earned* by the doctor. Know the difference between faith and blind faith. Faith is earned by the physician, not divinely bestowed upon him. It comes from showing concerned, competent and responsible care. Most do a competent job most of the time. However, too many factors get stirred into the pot to make the equation as a simple as "professionals = quality."

What are some of the nitty-gritty outpatient issues with which you'll be dealing? Some involve special situations such as mental health problems, chronic illnesses, undiagnosable conditions, and being considered a "bad" patient. These will be dealt with in later chapters. Here, we'll take a more general look at care during a generic or "plain vanilla" office visit. In the process, we'll follow a patient from start to finish.

Obviously, there can be a number of different circumstances surrounding a doctors appointment. It can be a first visit to a new doctor with the possibility of establishing a long-term professional relationship. It can be a return visit to a long-trusted physician, or it can be one of those more or less "catch-as-catch-can" visits to whomever is available in a group practice or convenience ("doc in a box") setting. This chapter will essentially assume the first scenario (a first visit), but many similar characteristics run through them all.

. . .

How do you select a doctor? What *type* of physician and then which physician in particular? Physicians are generalists or specialists. Unfortunately, which is which keeps changing. When I started out in practice in the late 1960s, internists and pediatricians were specialists. Now they're not; they're primary care physicians—

essentially generalists.

I've not been pleased with either the performance of, or the continuing trend to, family practice. Admittedly, this is my bias. But it's largely based on my own experiences in that kind of practice.

The generalist theory is a good one: Train practitioners to look at the "big picture" (the whole patient, including in the context of the family). Teach them to do most of the work, but refer patients to specialists for what the generalists don't know.

The problem? A lot of family physicians basically see children and adults for purely "medical" problems—avoiding both surgery and obstetrics. So they essentially function as pediatricians and internists without the proper training. They often haven't the time or skill to look at the "whole patient." In today's managed care environment, the family practitioner may be more of a "gatekeeper" (often keeping the gates closed rather than open) than a personal physician. He or she can make it more difficult to get needed specialty care. Yet more expensive—but specialized—care can save money in the long run. Decisions may be made not on the basis of "what's best for the patient," but rather "what's best for the patient compared to what's best for the practice."

Perhaps most important, it's hard to know what you don't know. If the doctor doesn't know that there are newer or alternative diagnostic approaches or treatments available, how would he know to refer for them? He'd have to refer everyone!

I think it would be quite possible—and valuable—for family physicians to redefine their roles so as to function as "personal medical advisors": Counselors who help in the prevention of illness and who serves as caregivers for more minor problems. But I don't see this happening in the near future.

If you decide that a family physician isn't your best choice, to whom should you turn? It's fairly simple. Children can see the pediatrician. Adults can see the internist and/or O.B.-Gyn physician as appropriate. In rural areas, where choices are more limited, the patient may not have the luxury of this kind of selection.

There, family doctors, physicians' assistants or nurse practitioners may be the best option.

. . .

Once the type of physician is chosen, how do you pick a specific doctor? Use as much available information as possible. Comments from current and previous patients can be very helpful. Be wary of 800 phone numbers offering referral services: They're likely to have their own agendas, such as shunting patients to a specific hospital. If you personally know any nurses, talk to them. They are unequivocally (to my mind, anyway) the best-informed source of advice regarding physicians. Nurses who work with a doctor in a hospital or office know what he or she is really like—blemishes and all.

Known facts regarding physicians—such as having had a lengthy practice in the same community or being board-certified—can be useful if you've nothing else to go on. Certification means that, after residency training, physicians have passed additional voluntary testing. But this is no guarantee of superior care. There are many excellent physicians who are not certified—and some certified ones you wouldn't want to see.

Be aware that there are directories available with factual information and even ratings of some, but not all, physicians. You can ask the librarian at your local public or medical library to help you find them. But ratings of even the best doctors at the best hospitals can be very subjective. And you can pay a high price financially, emotionally, and logistically, for going out of your own area to seek out the "best."

. . .

With name in hand, it's time to decide on the value and practicality of an appointment at this time. Unless the examination is for early detection (Pap smear, routine physical, and so on), don't assume that the visit may lead to the cure of anything. In fact it could be just the opposite.

One of my favorite sayings applicable to the purpose of health care goes something like this.

"To cure rarely, to relieve often, to comfort always."

For example, note the illnesses physicians frequently see for control rather than cure: hypertension, arthritis, diabetes, epilepsy, some chronic diseases of the heart and lungs. Add the problems that are—or can be—terminal, especially AIDS and cancer. Add to these the problems that usually get better largely by the body's own recuperative powers: colds, sprains, acne. Continue with problems we haven't had much success with, such as obesity and alcoholism.

Keep going with preventative care. Throw in the performance of cosmetic surgeries. Toss in unnecessary surgeries. Cesarian sections, hysterectomies, and tonsillectomies have a history of extensive overuse. Finally, consider all the vague, ill-defined, or transient symptoms for which no correct diagnosis is even made.

It's clear that we don't often cure. That's not to say we shouldn't value prevention, relief, and comfort. To comfort may be one of the most wonderful expressions of medical or any other kind of care. Just remember, all this is simply to say: Be realistic; you probably won't be going to the doctor for a cure.

. . .

In fact, there may be many actions *you* can take which may lessen your problem in more effective ways. Can A.A. (Alcoholics Anonymous) or simple determination control drinking? What about eating less and walking more to reduce weight? Might your problem be better handled by an optometrist, podiatrist, dentist, or psychologist? Many people report help from chiropractors after M.D.'s have failed to help their back pain. What about self-help books, better nutrition, and health food? And don't forget plain old *patience*—tincture of time. If you really need to see a doctor, you should do so—but take a comprehensive look at your other options as well.

. . .

So the doctor has been selected and you think it's worthwhile to see him—limited expectations not withstanding. As you start to think about phoning, it's time to put practical strategies in motion.

The process of making a medical appointment isn't as simple as making one for an oil change or haircut. This is a golden opportunity to actually start taking control. Be organized even before you make the call. Know what dates you have available (look far ahead on your calendar, just in case). Be ready to give a very brief description of the reason for the visit—general check-up, chronic headaches, breast lump, depression, introductory visit to just meet the doctor, have a specific type of examination form filled out, and so on.

If the reason for the visit is confidential, you don't have to share it with the receptionist. However, don't count on getting very far with, "it's personal." You may get the response, "I have to have something specific." You could reply with a general symptom you've been having instead of saying it's "for impotence," or "I think I have AIDS."

When you call, ask to speak with the doctor or ask for a return call. You'll probably get neither, but the response you receive will at least be informative in a limited way (even laughter from the receptionist tells you something). Your request for direct communication may be quite reasonable. For instance, you may wish to know his or her view on prescribing a new treatment you read about in the paper; you may be interested in trying it.

Find out if you'll actually see the doctor whose office you're calling. You might wind up spending most of the time with the physician's assistant, nurse practitioner, resident, or medical student. Ask how long a time slot is being reserved for you. You may have a 3 p.m. appointment for a very complicated problem. But has ten minutes or one hour been allocated? Ask! If it doesn't seem long enough, ask for more time. Most patients don't know how long their appointment time is, but the staff sure does.

Discuss fees. For the kind of appointment you're making, what is the usual charge? What is the expected method and timing of payment? These issues are much more easily handled in advance.

Inquire regarding practical issues about which the receptionist may or may not volunteer information. Are there routine forms to be filled out prior to actually seeing the doctor? Are parking facilities available (and accessible, if you are handicapped)? If appropriate, ask if providing specimens, such as urine, will be necessary.

After you make your appointment, you should attend to a variety of practical matters which will facilitate your visit. Be sure you have time available for whatever waiting may be necessary and for any testing that might be done following the meeting with the doctor. He or she may request X-rays, an electrocardiogram, or blood work. Often these can be scheduled in the near future, at a more convenient time for you. In some instances, it's appropriate to see if these can be done in advance of your appointment.

It may be valuable to bring any pertinent old records or X-rays. If circumstances warrant, request these from your prior physician in advance and bring them to the office. Don't delay your care by having the new doctor say "I can't tell you much more until we write for the old records" (and finally get them in perhaps a month or two). This adds to your cost and takes more of your time. Preferably, have the records sent to you rather than the new physician. Then make the decision as to whether or not to actually leave them with the office. You may want them again without the time and expense of another request or further copying.

Be sure to dress for both convenience and appropriate appearance. Doctors often consider women whose mode of dress might be considered dramatic or colorful as hysterical. Men who come resembling the current grunge look don't score points either. And people who come in with multiple layers of clothing, lots of snaps and hooks, and tightly encumbering garments pose an obstacle to the smooth flow of the examination.

The Waiting Room

A doctor's reception area isn't called a waiting room for nothing. Having a brief 10 or 15 minute delay, or on the very rare occasion having a major delay (if the doctor has a true emergency) is probably acceptable to most of us. But I feel strongly that regularly experiencing a 30-minute to 2-hour delay is just blatantly rude. Doctors and their staffs should know their practices better than to let this happen.

Unnecessary delays are inconsiderate and disrespectful of the patients. There are two root causes for such tardiness. First, more than ever, medicine is getting to be more like a business—and a poorly run one at that. Secondly, physicians have lost some of their professional and humanitarian anchors: They see such boorish behavior as their right. I've stopped buying the doctor shortage excuse as an acceptable explanation.

Here are a few of the "strategies" that patients can use to reduce their waiting.

1. Phone about an hour prior to the appointment. If the doctor is "running late" or has had an "emergency," ask for a revised time.

2. In the event that you need to see a number of physicians in a clinic, try to bunch the appointments together. As in the airline industry, the office staff should try to see that "on-time connections" are made.

3. When you initially make the appointment, ask the receptionist to suggest a day of the week and a time of day when the doctor typically runs on schedule. (He or she might routinely start on time at 9 a.m.—and then fall steadily behind.)

4. Tell the office to mail you in advance any registration

forms or special patient-completed questionnaires you can do at home.

If long waits are the rule rather than the exception with a particular doctor, be assertive in telling the receptionist and doctor that occasional emergencies are one thing, but routine extensive delays are another. You can also consider alternatives. See a specialist rather than a generalist in order to try to avoid unnecessary return visits. Switch to a doctor who is more considerate of patients or less busy. Or make appointments with non-physicians such as nurse-practitioners, or psychologists.

When you arrive at the office, ask if there will be a delay. If there will be one, ask how long. Office staffs usually have more information than they volunteer. They probably can tell you if you'll have an hour's wait. Tell them you'll be back—and go use the time for shopping, walking, or chores. This at least sends a subtle message of your inconvenience—if not displeasure. Just confirm that they're not going to cancel your appointment if you leave for a while.

I'm sure that some of these comments about scheduling won't be warmly received by all physicians, but I stand by them. Certainly, arguments could be made against just about any of these suggestions in particular cases. However, if one wants to decrease one's time in doctors' waiting rooms over a lifetime, I'd suggest giving them strong consideration.

A short wait can actually have some advantages for you. It gives you a chance to size-up the doctor's organization from the perspective of the waiting room. Listening to comments made by other waiting patients who are veterans of that practice can be very enlightening. Or you can engage them in conversation and subtly debrief them. From the time you check in until the time you are called to be seen, does the receptionist treat you and the other patients with courtesy and consideration?

Much information about the doctor and his practice can be gleaned simply by looking around the office, talking with the staff, or picking up printed materials. Where was the doctor trained? Is he board-certified? Is the practice solo or group? Can you talk to him personally on the phone or only via intermediaries such as nurses or receptionists? What are his fees? Which hospitals are used? Who covers his practice when he's unavailable?

Some areas might best be heard from the doctor himself: Does he have particular areas of interest and expertise within his field? What options does he allow for choice of hospitals if inpatient care is needed? And, is he open to getting second opinions if requested? Who are some of the consultants he might choose to use in the future in your case? If you call in with new symptoms and wish to be seen that day, is an appointment likely to occur? If you're really daring, ask about his philosophy of care or his personal philosophy of life. After all, this is a person to whom you are literally entrusting your life.

This can also be the time to review and re-evaluate the attitude you wish to project during your appointment: pleasant, prepared, open, informed, "professional" in approach, reliable, inquisitive, and interested—and wanting to be *involved.* These attributes might tick off a doctor who is used to passivity. You might even get the brush-off, or subtly but unconsciously be given substandard care. If you perceive these things happening, consider changing doctors.

The Examination Room

In a crowded waiting room, it's unlikely that the staff will come to your chair and quietly inform you that the doctor is ready to see you. More likely, a nurse holding your chart will call out to the assemblage, "Mary Smith!" Take it as a call-to-arms. Get ready to be as assertive as necessary in the service of your own best care.

If you are ushered fully dressed into a consulting room with comfortable chairs and a pleasant atmosphere in order to have a preliminary discussion, you are in the definite minority. More likely, you will be escorted to an examination room, given a gown of paper or minimum cloth, told to change and to wait because the doctor will be with you "shortly"—which may or may not be true. You may be told to "take everything off," not because it's necessary, but simply because it's easier for the staff to give such a general order rather than to tailor the amount of undressing to the particular need of that visit.

Finally, as if from stage left, the doctor cometh. Physicians differ in their initial approach to a patient. You may get some brief social chit-chat. The more minimalist approach is, "Hi, Mary, I'm Dr. Jones. What's wrong today?" This is the beginning of the interview or the "history" part of the exam in medical parlance. (For really sharp physicians this is also simultaneously the beginning of the "physical." Although no instruments are used, the exam has begun with careful observation of the appearance, mannerisms, and speech of the patient.)

The doctor's introduction as given above may imply the following: (1) "We are not equals," (2) "I am very important—and don't forget it," (3) "You are broken and need to be fixed by me," (4) "I have no time to waste; let's get down to business," and (5) "Speak when spoken to and be prepared to follow my orders." (Physicians quickly learn to be sparse in their speech.)

If you are a woman, you have about as much chance of having some psychological issues (even those relating to physical problems) fully understood by many male doctors as would an alien from outer-space. But, if you've come this far, do the best you can. I wouldn't waste a lot of the time trying to help the doctor understand how it feels for you to be naked for the exam, discuss menstruation, or explore issues of pregnancy or your sexuality, for example.

Although the doctor calls you "Mary" or "Bill," don't expect to be offered the opportunity to address him or her by first name. The common belief may be that he or she is putting you at ease; more likely, it's an assertion of dominance. I prefer formal titles for both parties. Being a physician is no guarantee of having the people skills necessary to put others at ease. You may even have to help the doctor to feel comfortable with you.

This is an ideal time to remind yourself of the issues of structure and time constraints. The doctor will certainly be ready with his or her structure to move you along—and, ultimately, out! After all, he or she knows the script perfectly. You should be prepared with your own structure to slow down the visit if necessary. To some extent, the patient needs to be manager of both the visit and the doctor. You want the biggest, most useful, and most healing bang for your buck. If the doctor fails to address all the pertinent issues, at least you should be prepared to do so.

So now the doctor has asked about the reason for your visit. It may be helpful to realize that a medical history is composed of a number of parts. They are all there for a reason. Every doctor may not cover every part on every visit. And there certainly is tremendous variation in how doctors take a history. But if you realize that a significant part of a history is lacking in your records or during the interview, you should volunteer the information on your own.

Here's a partial outline of a history, with an explanation of the purpose of each section:

- Chief complaint: This is the primary reason for the visit. It tells the doctor why you're there. It's usually some variation of "Why have you come?" or "What's the problem?"

- The history of the present illness: Provides details regarding the chief complaint. It allows the doctor to start sorting out the reason for your headache, fever, or vomiting, for example, from all the other possibilities.

- The past history: This gives additional clues to the diagnosis and it provides information on possible treatment approaches. It will include information such as previous illnesses and surgeries, the medication you're taking as a result of these, and the allergies or other serious reactions to medicines you've taken.

- Personal history: Tells the physician about your work, your family situation, your interests—all areas that could provide additional clues regarding diagnosis or treatment. Don't expect that much time will be spent on this section.
- Review of systems: A survey of various symptoms which may or may not seem to be related to the immediate situation, but can give further clues to diagnosis. Typically, you might be asked something like this: "Any headaches, sore throat, chest pain, difficulty breathing, nausea, vomiting, weight loss, abdominal pain, bowel changes?" and so on. Women may be asked about the possibility of a current pregnancy during this time. (And if you see the doctor write that you're "S.O.B," it means you're "short of breath.")

These sections of the history all make up pieces of a puzzle, which, when put together with a physical exam (possibly with other tests, X-rays, and even consultations with other physicians) can give a fuller picture of your health. And they'll set the stage for appropriate treatment recommendations.

About the *worst* possible responses for a patient to make during a history is saying either "It's in my records" or, "I already told that to Nurse So-and-So." In both the hospital and office, patients often find themselves being asked for information already recorded or told to others. Some of this repetition is due to inefficiency in the system. But often the repetition is necessary and useful.

Different professionals need a different perspective on the same information. A nurse may ask you about your medications simply to complete a form and provide preliminary information to the physician. The physician may need more detailed and specific prescribing information.

The doctor must clearly understand your current use of medications. The medications might be causing the symptoms of which you're complaining or they may have to be modified because of your new diagnosis. There may be an interaction between your current medications and any new prescriptions which might be given. If you're not also asked about over-the-counter medications, mention any that you are using.

It's understandably frustrating for doctors when patients have no idea what medications they are taking. "Two red ones at night and a green one twice a day—I don't know what they're for." This sort of ignorance is to the detriment of both patient and doctor. At the very least, bring your medications to the office in their labeled pharmacy bottles. (If you've filled out the medication section of the health care form in Appendix B of this book and brought it with you, you are ahead of the game.)

The doctor may simply wish to confirm that the recorded information is, indeed, correct and current. With some information, the *manner* in which it is conveyed can be more important than the information itself. The nurse may mark "divorced" on your office form. But the physician may note the anxiety or tears when inquiring about marital status.

When questions are presented, be concise in your answers. No matter how much you want to include every detail from your past, resist the urge. When your appointment is for the flu, the doctor does not want to hear, "Well, ever since I was a child, it's been one thing after another with my health. My mom was the same way. She was a really fascinating woman. So were my sisters..." Neither does he wish to know that a pain was "like a sharp spear thrown with lighting quickness by an Amazon warrior..." Learn to be brief, yet thorough.

You should be prepared to give a clear, concise answer regarding the chief complaint, incorporating some time frame if possible: "I've had stomach pains for three months," or "I'm here for a routine exam and have no current problems," or "I've been depressed for a year." There is nothing wrong with having rehearsed this. When clearly put, your response really helps the physician to help you.

This is also the time to answer a question which the doctor

will rarely ask: "Regardless of the problem, what do you want to get out of this appointment?" Be clear on what you expect: a second opinion on a diagnosis, a different treatment approach, a look toward possibly switching doctors, a one-time visit for a specific problem, or whatever.

While you make clear both your problem and your expectation(s) for the visit, I'd like to think that a really good doctor will essentially keep quiet for a while. With minor comments ("Go on") or just a nod, he or she will encourage you to provide as many of the salient details as you can remember before interrupting. Such an unintrusive approach avoids the possibility of prematurely introducing his or her preconceptions and biases.

Your comments may be followed by clarifying questions such as, "How would you describe the pain?" or "How has your appetite been?" I generally prefer to see the doctor ask questions in an open-ended fashion, such as, "Tell me about your sleep," rather than, "Are you having trouble sleeping?"

More personal questions sometimes make patients uncomfortable. When appropriate, physicians are supposed to ask questions regarding sexuality. If you're in the office for birth control, for example, it's certainly understandable to be asked about the frequency of intercourse. Certain symptoms might bring a question as to the specifics of sexual activity. I tell my medical students to at least introduce the issue of sex in almost every comprehensive examination. This can be done in a very general and non-threatening way: "Have you had any concerns regarding sexual functioning?" or (more open-endedly), "Are there any sexual issues you'd like to discuss?" If nothing else, such inquiries give the patient the message that the doctor is open to—and unthreatened by—sexual material. The patient learns that he or she can bring it up without embarrassment at a future visit.

I ask any female of potentially child-bearing years—married or not—if there is a possibility of pregnancy. While this question may sound sexist, it's extremely important for a number of reasons.

Pregnancy could possibly explain symptoms. And, diagnostic X-rays or certain medications might cause injury to the unborn child.

A good doctor may also ask questions which give you an opening to bring up a difficult subject. For example, he or she might say, "Sometimes when people get depressed, they think of injuring themselves. Have you had thoughts of suicide?" A question such as, "Symptoms like this sometime come from an illness picked up while traveling. Have you been out of the country recently?" may also prompt you to share information that you previously thought was unrelated to your problem.

. . .

So far, the doctor and patient have been trying to diagnose each other: The doctor is looking for the cause of the patient's problem. The patient is evaluating the doctor's competency, professionalism, and humanity. But can a patient evaluate a doctor's clinical abilities?

You can at least get some additional clues during your visit. There's probably some aspect or another of health care of which you already have a reasonable knowledge: Your own known illnesses, or the side effects or drug interactions of one of your medications. Ask the doctor about one of these. ("Is there anything I should know about my blood pressure medicine?") As you can always use more information, you can ask with straight face. See what sort of a response you get in terms of the information itself and the manner in which it's delivered. Was this—and other questions—answered fully and understandably?

. . .

Embarrassed by any of the questions? Don't be. First of all, it should all be pretty routine to the physician and staff. Secondly, the truly embarrassing things in our lives seem that way to us infinitely more than they do to anyone else. If the doctor does seem embarrassed, then I'd say it's his or her problem, not yours.

So be open. But don't be surprised if you feel that you can't "let it all hang out" the first visit. Good doctors realize this. There's nothing wrong with saying, "There's more, but I'm still a little uncomfortable. Perhaps we could talk about it at a future appointment." When the physician feels that the information may be crucial at the time, he or she can help you discuss it more comfortably.

If the going gets tough during the interview, it may help to recall what motivated your visit in the first place. It was probably fear, pain or suffering, hope for a long life, or the desire to survive. All are strong reasons to persevere in the face of discomfort.

If bringing brief notes in to the visit helps you convey your message, do so. The doctor won't necessarily appreciate this, wanting you to cut to the heart of the matter. He or she may see the notes as unnecessary baggage—and an obstacle to efficiency. It might be best to keep the notes to a few important points you want to be sure are included.

. . .

Now the physical examination can begin (although some doctors may combine the formal history with the formal examination, asking about allergies and symptoms as they look into your ears and feel your belly). The extent of the physical examination is dictated by the nature of the problem, the expectations of the patient, available time, and the habits and conscientiousness of the physician. "I twisted my ankle" takes a lot less time to check out than "I've lost weight" or "I feel tired." Or, if the patient is requesting a second opinion on an unresolved problem, the exam may take more time than usual.

A routine physical is a very special case—it has as many meanings as there are doctors. The actual time spent with the physician could be anywhere from two minutes to two hours. Unless most of the body's orifices are explored and most of the body's surfaces are touched—or at least looked at—the routine physical exam may be inadequate.

Exact guidelines are difficult to give. If you're a man, a rectal exam and genital exam will likely be included in any such comprehensive look. If you're a woman, anticipate a Pap smear and a pelvic and breast exam in addition to the other routine checks. I guess that the most reasonable yardstick would probably be this: If you don't feel you were adequately examined, you probably weren't. I'd estimate that the hands-on part of a reasonably thorough general physical should take a minimum of 10 to 15 minutes (more if a pelvic exam is included). People would be amazed at how much information physicians can gather in relatively little time.

. . .

Any exam, of course, should be done with respect, gentleness, and with regard to comfort, dignity, and modesty. A nurse in attendance during the examination of a female patient by a male physician can be a helpful addition, but I'm reluctant to say that this is necessary. Her presence is often more for the protection of the doctor if later there is some question of sexual impropriety, rather than for the patient's benefit.

During the exam, it's helpful if the doctor occasionally makes a comment on what to expect or on the nature of the findings. "This may be a little uncomfortable, but I'll go slowly," as he looks into your orifices. A word that the heart and lungs sounded "just fine" can be very reassuring as the examination progresses; ask how the exam is progressing if information isn't offered.

Since the doctor is now actually touching your body, issues of sexual appropriateness are introduced. Was there excessive or prolonged touching? Did the exam seem to go beyond the nature of the complaints? Was some sort of even very informal consent obtained prior to genital examination? Or was there an explicit or implied understanding in advance that it was going to be included? Without any registration of an objection by the patient, the physician might take silence as a consent. If you're concerned about certain aspects of the exam, say so. It can be difficult for a patient to distinguish the appropriate from the inappropriate. On the other hand, did the doctor even touch the *area* of concern in order to examine it?

. . .

Judgment time is now at hand—and I mean that literally. If the special expertise of physicians could be summed up in one word, it would be judgment. This is what all the preceding events have lead up to. On a practical level, this is what you are really paying for. The physician sifts through all the accumulated data: what you said, the records provided, and what the examination revealed. He measures this against all the lectures he has ever attended, all the textbooks he has ever read, all the patients he has ever seen, then he mixes in common sense and perhaps even intuition. He comes to a conclusion—a *judgment* if you will—of what all this means.

Then, from the near-infinite number of options available both diagnostically and therapeutically, he chooses what most reasonably seems to fit you and your needs. This is what you have come for.

Ideally, the doctor will give you a brief summary of the entire process. When an actual problem has been discovered, that summary might be similar to "This is what you told me. This is what I found. Based on my expertise, this is the conclusion I've drawn. Most likely, your problem is this. Here is what that means. Here's my recommendation and some alternatives. These are the pluses and minuses. This is the likely outcome. We can work together on this problem if you wish. Do you have any questions?" Or it might include a statement like, "It would be important to do some testing to confirm or identify the problem. Here's what I'd suggest."

If you don't hear something similar to the above scenario, you can introduce your own questions: "What did you find? What's your diagnosis? What do you recommend? Why?"

There are also a number of "generic" questions you can always have ready after the physician makes his pronouncements:

- Can you explain that in simpler terms?
- Can you explain that in greater detail?
- What are the possible complications (of the medicine, testing, or treatment procedure)?
- What are my options? (Or, tell me more about my options.)
- What else could it be?
- Are there physicians or centers specializing in this problem?
- What is the likely outcome?

It's a lot of information to take in. Good physicians will usually encourage questions on any points you might wish clarified or re-explained. Simple drawings, plastic models, or printed material relevant to the discussion are often used. Especially common these days—and to be encouraged—are printed medication instruction sheets. These can provide discussions of such issues as side effects, as well as other medications to avoid with the prescription. But the written material should rarely, if ever, completely take the place of a verbal discussion with the doctor.

If you're still confused, be assertive in getting a clarification. If you're not getting an adequate response, there may be a number of explanations. I think the basic cause is that physicians just don't allow enough time for appointments—to do so might not be "cost-effective." Or they may rely too heavily on printed material. Sometimes the doctor really may not know much beyond his or her previous comments and would feel threatened by questions.

. . .

In simple situations—especially with a satisfactory patient-doctor relationship—it may be possible to wind things up right here. You understand and agree to a treatment program which is recommended for a limited time due to limited illness. Ideally, you get better and have no treatment complications.

In very complicated and serious cases, however, no decision may be called for right at that moment. Don't feel pressured if the situation is not truly an emergency. Instead, a discussion limited to the findings, prognosis (probable outcome), and options may be warranted. Before or during a return visit (without unnecessary delay), a decision can be made. Hopefully this is after some study and careful reflection by you. A second opinion may be an important part of the process.

Even in some less difficult situations, the doctor may suggest a return visit. Or, if a successful outcome is likely, the doctor may suggest that you return only if necessary. In any case, you should probably be informed that a return visit or call would be welcome at any time.

During this wrap-up is a time to continue to exercise your control and responsibility over your care. Don't leave if you feel dissatisfied or confused; tell the doctor what your concern is.

I have a fantasy about the above information-sharing process. Someday, the doctor will give the patient a written report of all the pertinent material as a supplement to the discussion—not just a pre-printed medication instruction sheet.

The form might look something like the one on page 157.

As a final consideration, remember: Doctors usually don't offer a guarantee for their treatment plans, nor should they. Medical practice is still an art, not a science. No treatment is assured of working without any possibility of complications.

. . .

To fully understand the dynamics of an appointment, a look at the visit from the doctor's perspective is also in order. It's helpful to be aware that the visit—especially with a first-time patient—

Doctor's Report

Date of visit: ______________________

Chief complaint: ______________________

Any important finding on examination: ______________________

____

Formal name of diagnosis: ______________________

What that means: ______________________

The primary recommendation is: ______________________

____

Advantages of this recommendation: ______________________

____

Disadvantages of this recommendation: ______________________

____

Alternatives and why are they not the primary recommendation: ______________________

____

Medication instructions and side effects: ______________________

____

The next appointment: ______________________

Problems which may arise prior to the next scheduled appointment, for which a call would be indicated: ______________________

____

____

may be very difficult for the physician. The clinical visit is actually a very complex encounter. The doctor has many tasks to perform. While I'm not necessarily suggesting that this sequence, or even each part, is necessary with every visit; here's a generic list of the doctor's agenda:

- Provide an introduction
- Make the patient feel at ease
- Make a positive impression (after all, the doctor's only human too)
- Evaluate the patient's financial ability and general reliability (he would like to get paid and have instructions followed)
- Verify the patient's consent, even informally
- Take an adequate history (more likely to be "focused" these days, rather than inclusive)
- Select and perform the appropriate examinations
- Review previous records
- Review lab/X-ray findings
- Look at the patient as a whole (a "bio-psycho-sociocultural" approach)
- Come up with an appropriate diagnosis and perhaps some additional possibilities (called "rule out" or "differential diagnosis")
- Explain findings, recommendations, potential complications, and the likely prognosis
- Order the planned treatment, medications, testing, or referrals

- Provide useful written material
- Decide on and arrange for follow-up care
- Answer questions
- Interact with family if appropriate
- Document much of the above (for clinical and legal reasons, records must be kept)
- Determine and submit a fee
- Continually deal with logistical issues (getting the nurse in, the family out, the patient on the exam table, dealing with phone calls and other interruptions)
- Protective measures (called "CYA"—"cover your ass"—or "defensive medicine")

The appointment process is somewhat ritualized so that the doctor can get all this done. Understandably, physicians are annoyed when the patient adds at the end of the appointment: "And by the way, will you look at this..." Avoid pulling the appointment off the tracks. Concentrate on the reason given for the appointment in the first place. Or, ask the doctor at the beginning of the visit if there will be time for the additional concern.

. . .

Every patient poses a number of potential threats to the doctor. The most obvious example of this is the malpractice suit. Probably more common, but less obvious, is the threat to the doctor's ego. In fact, their egos may even be more vulnerable because they have been indoctrinated to believe in their superior position as an almost God-given right. Dissatisfaction from patients and families doesn't sit well with physicians.

There is a rarer and more serious threat to the doctor which seems on the increase. Doctors have been singled out in a number of ways for actual physical attack by patients and non-patients alike. Murders of physicians for reasons related to their practice—while not common—are certainly not unheard of. Attacks on physicians who perform abortions reveals only one aspect of this. It all points up, again, that doctors are human beings with both imagined and all-too-real worries.

. . .

The office visit can also involve a number of philosophical issues you should consider. High among these issues is a recognition of the limitations of modern medicine. What we don't know about the human mind and body would fill far more volumes than what we do know. Failure to recognize this reality results in unrealistic expectations by the patient and far too much unnecessary intervention by the practitioner. Patients may incorrectly feel they can beat a cancer, and the doctor may feel obligated to never stop trying to save their lives using science and technology. Ultimately, patients get discouraged and doctors get defensive.

There are also issues of cost-effectiveness. This is a word which is destined to be used more frequently as part of the vocabulary of clinicians, bureaucrats, and maybe even patients. After all, bureaucrats and insurers have only "X" number of dollars to spend. But the term "cost-effectiveness" may become largely irrelevant at the level of that individual, that single life.

There are many other issues which involve the patient-doctor relationship. Occasionally, there is the choice of being cared for by a pleasant but marginal physician versus an ornery but competent one. There is also the question of "doctor hopping," which physicians, in general, don't like (unless the hop is in their direction). But what is a patient to do when a problem is unresolved by a doctor who seems unapproachable with regard to options—or even for just further discussion?

There are significant moral and ethical issues you may wish to consider. Where do the responsibilities of the patient and the doctor begin and end (especially with regard to patients who don't follow treatment instructions, or who drink and smoke to their own detriment)? Where does the doctor stand on abortion, euthanasia, discontinuation of life-support? Does the doctor and office staff respect your confidentiality—or is this precept broken in practice as well as in spirit?

Obviously, selecting a physician involves more than selecting someone who is simply technically competent.

. . .

Finally, you must evaluate your office visit experience—and the doctor.

Test the situation by asking yourself these questions. Were you treated with respect and courtesy by the physician and other staff? Was the office environment reasonably comfortable and pleasant? Was the overall process (including making the appointment) efficient and productive? Were there a lot of interruptions such as phone calls and the doctor being called out of the room? Did you get the impression of competence, concern, and compassion? Did the doctor respect you as a full partner in your own care? Was there adequate time, especially to answer your questions? Were you heard? Were you allowed to become involved? Did you feel satisfied for having had the appointment? Was there a sense of any sexual inappropriateness? Was it money (or time and effort) well spent?

A pertinent question is: Did you get better? Or did you get adequate service if you were well to begin with? And if you did get better, was it because of, in spite of, or unrelated to your visit—or can you even tell?

If the doctor flunks your test, you have a number of options which will be discussed in Chapter Eighteen. If the doctor did well, this could be the start of a beautiful relationship. In this case, the process of bonding which can develop into a nurturing, trusting, and mutually beneficial patient-doctor relationship has already started. Over time, such an attachment can mean not only more knowledgeable care, but more "caring" care.

If you felt shortchanged and left feeling dissatisfied and unfulfilled due to many unanswered questions, then use what you've learned. Try again, either with the same physician (but using a more assertive approach), or consider going elsewhere.

You might have to go with your gut feeling. Ask yourself: "Am I comfortable with what just occurred?" Answering the rhetorical question "Would I recommend this doctor—this experience—to others?" may help. Better yet, ask if you felt like just another obstacle in the doctor's day, or did you feel like a partner working together toward a common goal—your health?

Keep in mind that disagreeing with the doctor, being unhappy with the conclusions and recommendations, or even having an unsatisfactory result are *not necessarily* indications of poor care. We pay physicians for their judgment. We ask them to be reasonable in their care. We can't always expect to be thrilled by the conclusions. We cannot even ask for or expect doctors to be unfailingly right. We only ask that they exercise good judgment, in patients' best interest, based on a competent and compassionate level of care.

. . .

Patients and the medical world must learn to work together in partnership. Make every possible effort to have your physician, and your office visits, be assets in your care—not further stumbling blocks. Establishing an ongoing and solid relationship with a personal physician can be a big part of having each visit count maximally. I certainly recommend such continuity as preferable to sporadic trips to see whichever physician happens to be available at the local "doc-in-a-box."

This has been a long chapter. But there's a good reason for it. At a crossroads of your life—perhaps at the moment of its greatest crisis—you and your doctor may need to stand together. I'd like you to understand as much as possible about this relationship—and to pick your "partner" as wisely as you can.

In the process, remember this rallying cry: "Involve me! It's *my* health."

CHAPTER 11

The Hospital Stay

Pearl:
When hospitalized, take little for granted: ask, check, verify, confirm.

Welcome to the medical world's version of "The Greatest Show on Earth"—the hospital stay!

Someday, almost everyone of us will be a hospital patient at least briefly. Although the overall length of stay has been shortened, the end result is simply that all the risks which are discussed throughout this book have been compacted into a shorter period of time. In addition, new risks, such as premature discharge and hurried care, can develop precisely because of the abbreviated stays.

Throughout your stay, you may feel about as welcome as an uninvited guest—and just about as comfortable. The traditional expectation of the hospital is that you lay low, say little, and stay out of the staff's way.

Actually, that type of approach could have some benefit for you. At a certain level, in dealing with routine problems, hospitals often do a pretty decent job if simply left to their own methods. Unfortunately, "often" isn't good enough.

I don't share my somewhat pessimistic view here to unduly frighten you. When you go to the hospital, the chances are overwhelming that you will get reasonably appropriate care and suffer no harm. But I think the system is capable of much more than giving you good odds; I believe it can give you excellent ones.

. . .

There are a number of ways of positively influencing the outcome—or at least the comfort—of a hospital stay. Come to the hospital both forewarned and forearmed. Ideally, you'll bring with you a solid knowledge of your illness (or at least some basic information about your symptoms). You should also know something about the treatments you've already had or are currently receiving.

Bring clothes that are appropriate for resting in your bed but still let you resemble a functioning human being. Sweats are a reasonable choice. If you think you're going to be up to it, bring plenty of business work or pleasure reading so that you don't vegetate unhappily in a bed all day. You have a life—continue to live it, whether you are in the hospital or not. And, finally, come with a mindset to be inquisitive and involved in your care.

A positive attitude can also be helpful. Come with the intention of being pleasant, informed, appropriately assertive, and friendly, not meek and submissive. However, don't count on staff admiration for your knowledge and efforts. These attributes may just as easily be seen by the staff as stumbling blocks in their efforts to get their individual jobs done. You are moving onto their turf. Be prepared to take a reasonable stance in your own best interest, even when that is not popular. The question you need to answer is, "How far am I willing to go?" or, even, "At what point will my assertiveness actually jeopardize my care?"

. . .

Perhaps the best way to demonstrate how to get the most from your stay would be to run through a fairly typical hospital stay. Throughout this example—and during your own actual hospital stay—you can use some of the information you learned in earlier chapters which discussed doctors, hospitals, nurses, and other members of the Biz-Med Complex. Preparation for a hospital stay should begin well in advance of the event—preferably even before the need for hospitalization has come up.

Where you are hospitalized will largely be a function of four factors: (1) where your health care plan allows you to be hospitalized, (2) where your doctor has privileges, (3) where any specialized services you need are available, and (4) last—and probably least—your own preference.

Obviously, it's important to read your insurance policy as well as talk with your doctor in regard to which facility will be available to you. Within a community, hospitals generally have better or worse reputations. Personal and family experiences, as well as information from friends and acquaintances, should also be considered in regards to hospital choice. Information on the number of beds, accreditation, special resources, and so on, is fairly easy to come by.

For certain kinds of problems, some hospitals have exceptional reputations. For instance, some are well known as diagnostic centers; others may be especially competent in heart surgery, burn care, or even hernia repair. There are pros and cons to seeking these out. The obvious pro is their expertise and success rate brought by repeated experience and practice with these problems. The downside is the additional travel and expense that may result, not to mention the fact that your insurance may not cover your choice. Perhaps even worse is being away from the love, support, and protection of family and friends. And, facilities with great public images still are no guarantee of quality care.

If the facility is associated with a medical school or other training institution, be aware that you may be used as part of the training. On the other hand, you are more likely to be on the cutting edge (no pun intended) of advanced technology and may be seen by residents who are backed up by some of the most experienced and senior attending physicians in the country. Your case is more likely to be considered by a number of different physicians—although you won't necessarily receive their individual input.

On the minus side, your care is more likely to be splintered among a number of providers. You're more likely to be just another case being run through an even more rigid and unyielding system than in a community hospital. Finally, a major portion of your direct medical care is likely to be provided by the most inexperienced members of the physician-team: the junior residents and medical students. If your admission is elective rather than an emergency, try not to schedule it for July when the new residents start their training. I'd suggest giving them a few weeks to figure things out.

At a minimum, when hospitalized in these academic facilities, know who your attending physician is, know which physicians are working under "the attending" in training positions, and know which are the ones who are acting as consultants. No matter how many doctors are involved in a patient's care, there should be only one in charge.

A clue to who you are dealing with in training facilities is provided by identification badges (which should be noted carefully), uniforms, and length of time spent with you. In general, the shorter the white coat or the more papers and implements stuffed in the pockets of these particular caregivers, the lower in the hierarchy they will be. Also, the longer time spent with you, the lower he or she is likely to be on the totem pole.

Trainees are often given too much access or responsibility, but, of course, this is how they learn. Despite their inexperience, you may feel more secure for having talked to someone—even a medical student—for an hour or so. This is probably much longer than your own physician is going to spend with you at any given time in the hospital.

People's titles aren't always accurate descriptions. Medical students are sometimes instructed to call themselves "Doctor" although they certainly do not qualify for this title. You, on the other hand, are more likely to be called "Bill" or "Susie" regardless of your age or standing in the community. You may occasionally be asked how you would like to be addressed. Don't think it is snobbish to respond "Mr. Smith" or "Ms. Jones" if that is your preference.

One final note about female medical students (and physicians, for that matter): They're likely to be just as hassled and worn down as their male counterparts, so don't necessarily expect an extra dose of "warm fuzzies" just because you are working with a female caregiver. They often have an even tougher job than their male counterparts. And don't assume that every woman in white you see is a nurse.

. . .

The time has come! The doctor informed you during an office visit that you require inpatient surgery or medical services too extensive for outpatient care. Arrangements have been made for your hospital stay. You have come to the hospital and found the admitting area. In staff parlance, you are about to become "the gallbladder in 523" or "the colitis in 801."

You can shorten your time in the admitting area if you come prepared. Have all of your health care policy information. Understand what sort of options your policy gives you in regards to a single or a double room. While everyone has their own preference, I'd certainly opt for a private room if it's feasible. There is enough psychic trauma that goes on in a hospital stay without having to deal with getting a new roomie. He or she may not be some quiet person who is just going to lay there. The other patient may be much sicker than you, with machines humming and beeping, and a long procession of visitors—not to mention health care providers—coming to the bedside. Groaning and snoring only complicate matters. This you can do without.

In admitting, you may be asked to sign a number of forms. I certainly wouldn't say that signing them is unimportant, but even a non-lawyer would seem justified to ask "How much legal weight can these have under the circumstances?" A long detailed form in small print may be handed with little if any explanation to a very ill person. This hardly seems to constitute informed consent to me. But a hospital attorney may well try to make such a case in a malpractice suit.

There is an oft-repeated misconception regarding entering a hospital. We frequently hear of someone who admitted himself or herself. This is often within the context of a sports or entertainment figure who is going into a drug treatment program. No one admits themselves—at least, not in my experience. Admission is upon a doctor's order. I think the misuse may attempt to convey a sense of power or control by the patient, or his/her publicist.

. . .

Once you are in your room, it's time to "nest" and get comfortable. My wife, Pat, who is an experienced nurse and an experienced patient, tells me that bringing the following items can make a hospital stay more comfortable: your own pillow; toiletries and tissues of *your* preference (the hospital may not use your brands); family photos and a few other personal items to "soften" the room; pen and note pad; reading material; loose, casual, comfortable clothing (sweats and T-shirts are ideal if appropriate to your clinical care requirements); non-slip slippers and socks; flashlight; small clock, small radio with personal headset; your dignity—and keep it close to you.

Don't be a slug who slips into a pair of pajamas (or worse, a hospital gown), robe and slippers, and hibernates in the room. Put on your sweats. If there is nothing scheduled following the admitting routine and your physical condition permits it, let the nurse know that you'll be around the hospital and will be checking back at some specific time. Be on your way to exploration—even if it's in a wheelchair. You're not being held prisoner; you're a patient. Go find out about your new environment.

Now, the staff could prevail by telling you that "Doctor could be here any time." But, if enough patients are this assertive, perhaps hospitals will start taking patients' time into consideration. Nurses often feel that you simply should sit in your room and wait for staff to visit at their convenience—not yours. For the first hour or two of admission this might be a reasonable approach. The nurse will certainly want to spend some time with you reviewing your history and getting some of the basic information needed to help in your care. But after that, professional visits and testing can be at irregular intervals and far between. Ask your nurse or the desk clerk at the nurses' station to find out when staff are expected to see you next or when testing will occur. Be cooperative and flexible, but you needn't feel like a hostage. If you go off the unit, let the staff know where you'll be.

Don't be an invalid if you are really not one. After getting guidance from the nurse, do for yourself what you can. Get yourself out of bed and into the bathroom for your shower or toilet. Dress yourself. Bring your own water pitcher out to the nurses station and ask if you can fill it. By the same token, if you need care, insist upon it. If the nursing staff seems overwhelmed, don't get angry at them. Request to see a supervisor and express your concern that the nurses appear to be carrying too large of a patient load.

Try to keep your life in the hospital as normal as possible. Stick to as many personal routines as circumstances allow. If you are able to get up and about and have no special dietary requirements, go to the cafeteria for some meals. Make sure you know where the gift shop and newspaper machines are located. Encourage visits by family and friends you would like to see. For patients so inclined, visits from the hospital chaplain can be both of practical assistance as well as philosophically or spiritually supportive.

Of course, the sicker you feel, the less active, independent and self-advocating you may be. This is where prior preparation can pay dividends. Do what you can before you are ill. When a serious illness has occurred, it's time to have as much information and outside support as you need. Families can be especially important at this time, but friends, minister or priest, or even your lawyer can help advocate for you if necessary.

Depending on circumstances, the only doctor who visits you during your hospital stay may be your own personal physician. Since he or she already knows your history and has examined you, this visit may be brief but be sure to utilize this time to its fullest. Keep track of what testing has been done and inquire as to the results when the physician comes in. Bring him or her up to date on the symptoms you're having and request an evaluation of your current situation or progress. If you are seen by members of the hospital staff, such as residents, they may be spending more time with you and review much of the same information as your doctor.

Just because your doctor doesn't spend much time at the bedside doesn't mean he or she is not spending time on your case. Reports from nurses, consultations with colleagues, review of charts and test results, and making notes in your record—all done out of your sight—can all take considerable time.

Being able to provide an accurate medical history in the hospital can be critical to your health. Doctors realize that a good history is still the most important part of the diagnostic process. But it's a dying art, taking more time and skill than ordering a high tech test. Knowledge of medications, previous problems, and allergies can be some of the more difficult areas for patients to recall in detail, particularly if they feel ill. You can use the "Brief Personal Medical History Form" in Appendix B to assist in this task. Complete it, photocopy it, and bring a number of copies with you. But don't just shove this into the face of an interviewer and say, "It's all here." Instead, provide it as a useful tool to help the person taking the history.

At a very minimum, know the drugs you were taking just prior to hospitalization, the dose, and frequency of administration. It helps to simply drop the bottles into a small bag before leaving home and bring them all with you.

Each time your doctor visits, find out what changes are being made in your program. Ask *why*. Ask what options might be available. Use an inquisitive, but friendly, manner. Don't accept too brief of answers or hurried replies. This is your health and life.

Ideally, your doctor will volunteer important information without prompting, including about your medications.

Each time you are to receive medication take a look at the pills and make sure that they are a part of what you recognize as your treatment program. If a nurse is giving you an injection or some medication via your I.V. (intravenous) equipment, be sure to ask what the medication is prior to receiving it as well as its general purpose. And, make an effort to have *all* your personal caregivers be able to recognize you by name and face, not just by wrist identification badge.

If you are sharing a room with another patient, confidential communication can certainly be a problem. Don't let the physician get away with the subterfuge of simply drawing the curtain between the two of you as if this will create an impenetrable sound barrier. If you feel the material to be discussed is sensitive, assertively tell the physician that, if at all possible, you would like to go to a more private place to discuss the issue.

This would be a good time to mention the value of having some reference materials in your room. At a minimum, I would suggest that you bring both a *Merck Manual* and a layman's medication guide (any number of these guides are available in bookstores). This book might be helpful as well.

Occasionally, your doctor may call in another consultant if he or she feels that there is a particular challenge to your case and wants further input. (Consultants are experienced physicians, usually specialists in other fields.) You may not always be aware in advance that there are plans to have a consultant involved. He or she may just bounce in one day, assuming that the patient has been prepared for the visit. As a psychiatrist, I've had this occur on a number of occasions—with the patient unwilling to proceed with the interview.

Generally, the consultant is well known to the physician who requests assistance. (Doctors don't usually ask their enemies to consult.) Don't be satisfied if the consultant says, "I will discuss this with your doctor" after completing the examination. You can at least request that the findings be discussed with you—now. Then the consultant can discuss any findings with your doctor. Of course, your request may or may not meet with success.

If you are having surgery, you will probably also be visited by a representative from the anesthesiology department. I say "representative" because it may not be the person who will actually do the work.

Ask if you might meet the person who will actually be administering the anesthetic. After all, anesthesia will be as important a part of your care as the surgery itself. And you—or your insurance company—will be paying the bill. Personally, I would much rather talk directly to the person who was going to anesthetize me, rather then someone who is simply filling out forms. (There's also an advantage to you in comfort as well. Being wheeled into an operating room can be traumatic experience. I'd like to see as many familiar people as I could.)

I realize that many people who are having surgery simply want to be "put to sleep," but this may not necessarily be the best solution. If clinically indicated, I would much prefer a local or regional anesthetic injection that would allow me to stay awake during the procedure. This would also avoid the complications of a more general anesthetic which affects the entire body. The selection of the type of anesthetic is certainly an area in which a patient might be given some input.

The person who handles this aspect of your care is likely to be either an anesthesiologist (who is a doctor) or an anesthetist (who is a nurse). I feel about these two the way I feel about psychotherapists and their credentials: The best ones aren't necessarily those with the most degrees. All things being equal, I would rather have my anesthesia administered by a physician. However, a good, competent nurse who will spend time with me pre-operatively and who appears generally competent would be acceptable as well. This is especially true if the surgery wasn't particularly complicated or I had no other current medical problems.

The final person you will want to meet is your surgeon. I'm told that in the old days there were "ghost surgeons" who came into the operating room after the patient was asleep, and left before he awoke. The patient would never see who actually did the work. I suppose the general practitioner could then take the credit.

If your own doctor isn't doing the surgery, you will want to meet with your surgeon prior to the operation (ideally, even prior to hospitalization). It is never too late to explore options regarding alternative approaches, getting a different surgeon, or even refusing the surgery if necessary. Certainly, all the significant complications of the surgery should be adequately explained to you in advance.

. . .

What happens when you actually arrive at the surgical suite? You'll probably see a minimum of four people in the room. One will be the person administering the anesthetic and monitoring your response to it (either the anesthesiologist or anesthetist). Another will be the surgeon. A scrub nurse wearing sterile attire assists the surgeon in many ways, including handing him or her instruments. The circulating nurse who is not "sterile" will bring additional materials into the room as necessary to provide them to the scrub nurse. Sometimes technicians are used in place of nurses.

Of course, surgeries are often fairly complicated these days and there may be any number of additional members of the surgical team. These may or may not be physicians. They may be additional nurses, surgical technicians, lab technicians, X-ray personnel, or even medical photographers.

If you know you will be awake during the surgery, ask in advance for the surgeon to keep you generally informed of what is happening. When you're awake, there isn't likely to be as much "table talk" amongst the surgical staff. This can result in better attention to the situation at hand. And be aware that the need to switch to a different form of anesthetic sometimes arises during the surgery. A surgery in which you start out awake may be one in which you wind up asleep as circumstances change.

. . .

If your doctor comments that he'll increase your personal comfort privileges (for example, permission to have a shower), promptly verify that this is passed along in writing to the nursing staff. One patient waited days for this to be communicated. Another didn't get the dietary increase her physician had promised. She simply picked up the phone and called the dietary department and told them to send up the appropriate tray. While I wouldn't necessarily recommend using this direct route, it was effective.

With each passing day of hospitalization, most patients find themselves doing better and better. Diagnostic issues are being clarified, symptoms are diminishing, suffering is decreasing. Discharge is happily looming in the near future. All seems well.

For some patients, unfortunately, this is not the case. They feel they are no better or are even worse. How can these patients intelligently evaluate their situation? And what options are available to them for making productive changes?

If treatment does not appear to be progressing satisfactorily, a number of possible causes arise: (1) the treatment is the best available, but the condition is unresponsive; (2) the physician is clinically incompetent or a poor "manager" of the case (doesn't take enough time, doesn't get appropriate consultations, and so on); (3) the hospital is inadequate to the task of providing appropriate staff or services; (4) the patient's expectations are unrealistic, or (5) some combination of the above.

How can a patient recognize if their care is satisfactory? Few single indicators are likely to be definitive. But you can begin by referring to the ten numbered points near the conclusion of Chapter Eight. (Also, refer to Chapter Eighteen on "Dissatisfaction with Care.")

If you decide you have a serious concern, here are some of your options: (1) have a heart-to-heart talk with your doctor and try to resolve the problem, (2) try to switch doctors, (3) request that a consultant follow along in your management, (4) request transfer to another part of the hospital if the problem seems to be due to the care on your particular unit or floor, or (5) request transfer to another hospital. Check your insurance to determine if some of these actions might affect your coverage. Additionally, you can request to talk with the nursing supervisor or use the patient hot line if one is available at your hospital.

When you take any of these actions, you're talking serious business. Proceed cautiously, perhaps bringing family or friends into the process. Ultimately, you have the authority to request any of the above. But your requests may not be honored.

If the hospital has a patient representative, contact him or her. This encounter could vary from extremely effective to absolutely ineffectual. This person could be one of your strongest allies, but be aware that he or she is most likely on the payroll of the hospital.

. . .

Let's assume that your stay has gone reasonably well and the time of discharge is at hand. Doctors used to keep people in the hospital until they were well. These days, patients often stay until they are just marginally able to go home. Many patients feel almost thrown out of the hospital. They sometimes have very uncomfortable and inconvenient recuperations at home or in a nursing facility, with an occasional need to return to the hospital due to a premature discharge. For example, one hears more and more about mothers and babies being sent home 24 hours or less after delivery.

If you feel that you are being shoved out, tell the doctor. Say that you really don't feel well enough to continue your care outside of the hospital and request a longer stay. If you are sent home anyway and feel that your discharge was handled inappropriately, certainly you can complain to your insurer if that is the party who was blamed for the early discharge. Of course, first I would verify it was at least in part due to the urgings of the insurer. If the insurance was provided by an employer, let that employer know what happened.

Remember that insurers don't *discharge* patients. They simply refuse to *pay* for any additional service. Formal complaints to regulatory bodies, or even legal action, are other potential options.

. . .

At the time of discharge, be sure that there is adequate opportunity to sit down with your physician and review the hospitalization. There may be medications that you will need to take following discharge. Be sure you not only have prescriptions, but that you understand what they are for. Be aware of any side effects and potential drug interactions. Make sure you fully understand all additional instructions regarding dressing changes, dietary information, exercise programs, and recreational and work limitations.

I feel that you almost certainly should also know your official diagnosis as it is listed in the hospital records—not that you had "a bug," "a tumor—we got it all," "stress," or something similarly vague. A diagnosis made in the hospital is more likely to be correct than one made in the office. This is because your physician has had the advantages of (1) seeing the illness over time, (2) getting reports from the staff who has had you under 24-hour a day observation, (3) greater availability of testing, (4) seeing what, if anything, was the response to treatment, and (5) dealing with a sicker patient who was likely to have more clearly defined findings.

Be sure you understand under which circumstances you are to contact your physician if there are problems in the meantime.

This may be a good time to let the physician know that you would appreciate a copy of the discharge summary for your personal health records. The discharge summary is the physician's account of your hospitalization. It contains extremely valuable information for your future reference, as well as material which may help your physicians years later. Not only that, but it may answer a lot of questions that are still a mystery to you with regard to the hospitalization. If you had surgery, ask for a copy of both the surgeon's operative report as well as the pathologist's report on any tissue that may have been removed.

Try to anticipate which visit from the doctor will be his or her last to you. It's amazing how quickly and easily doctors seem to slip away from the patient before all pertinent questions are addressed. Then, the role of the nurse becomes even more important in the discharge process.

. . .

From the time you are admitted to the time you are discharged, it can be very helpful if you keep a diary. In this, record not only what has actually happened during each day, but your own impressions of what occurred. Keep track of the tests you have had and of the information you have received from the doctor and other practitioners. Record in the diary any questions that come to you and explore these with the physicians when they visit.

If you feel that there were untoward incidents that occurred, be certain to record these in detail with the names of the people involved. This information can be used later at the level of an informational complaint to the hospital—or even in a lawsuit, if appropriate.

. . .

In summary, we cannot do without hospitals; but we can do without their often inefficient, uncaring, ineffective, and even dangerous ways. Your entrance into the hospital is no time to lose your sense of empowerment within the medical world. Remain informed, alert, and inquisitive. More than ever, this is also the time to say, "Involve me! It's *my* health."

CHAPTER 12

"Public Sector" Care

Pearl:

As you take your place in the health care arena, be especially cautious if you're sitting in the public sector "tier."

In many people's minds, "public sector" care conjures up an image of inadequate services, inefficient systems, unresponsive practitioners, and poor quality care. Many times this picture is fairly accurate. However, it's very important to distinguish between the caregivers and the administrators who try, and the caregivers and administrators who don't. This same variability of attitude can be noted between different systems and individual facilities themselves.

What happens in public facilities is frequently a reflection of our society's priorities—and often a stain upon our values. There may be a number of reasons which could be used to justify the existence of a public sector. Who would deny that a major reason these institutions continue today is that they are generally seen as a cheaper way for taxpayers to support care for the poor (and powerless)? Ironically, it's probably *more* expensive to subsidize such substandard and inefficient care.

The existence of the public sector also provides the opportunity for those with some specific social agendas to promote them. For example, if largely unrestricted sexual activities are to be seen as a national "standard," public sector services can allow for the implementation of that standard as well as the management of the consequences.

Regardless of the reason(s) for its existence, the end result is the same: Public sector care runs the risk of allowing society to abandon its outcasts and unfortunates while posing as their protectors.

. . .

It's actually somewhat difficult to even define the term "public." Would you include VA hospitals where not all the public is eligible for care and the patients can be seen as having earned their benefits? What about non-governmental facilities funded by charities and private donations? I would at least exclude military hospitals for active duty personnel. These latter facilities fulfill a specific need probably unattainable within the private sector, especially during times of armed conflict.

So, I'll paint with a broad stroke here and simply define public sector care as essentially *not* private sector care. That is, these are facilities where money and insurance are not the major keys for entrance by the patient. Examples would be county hospitals, state mental health facilities, free community outpatient clinics, and many other facilities.

Private versus public systems has also been described as "two-tiered," i.e., two levels of care. One is generally for those who have resources and the other is for those don't.

Sometimes the tiering is excused as occurring on the surface only. These facilities are said to perhaps lack some of the conveniences or pleasantries of the private sector, but to deliver the same quality of care. Having trained and worked in more of these facilities than I can literally even recall, I'll tell you it just isn't so. The quality is very often lower—sometimes *much* lower.

Exceptions to poor quality were alluded to above. This chapter is not intended to criticize all staff or all administrators of public facilities. They are often efficient, effective, and well-intentioned. They may work valiantly, providing the only services available to some people. Nor is it to be critical of all these facilities. Some do at least an adequate job and a few are even outstanding. For example, the burn unit at Cook County Hospital in Chicago has been said to be a national leader in treatment of burn patients. And, many public sector emergency rooms are probably better prepared to handle a patient with severe trauma than many private facilities.

Keeping in mind that there are exceptions, it's best not to lose sight of the forest for the trees: "public sector" generally implies substandard care in an inefficient environment.

I once saw a fascinating example of public sector waste. A workman came into a doctor's office and perfunctorily stuck a colored dot on everything with an electric cord. Seeing this, I was curious and made an inquiry as to his task. I was told (without a hint of embarrassment) that it was a requirement that such electrical equipment needed to be periodically certified as safe. I didn't personally check the regulation, but I guess it read that "colored dots should be regularly stuck on electrical devices" and not that "following careful testing, colored dots should be stuck on electrical devices which prove to be safe."

A system of public facilities is "valuable" in three ways. From a practical standpoint, care *must* somehow be provided to the poor who often don't have adequate access to care provided in the private sector. Second, by providing these facilities we can say with a clear conscience that "we've done our part." If the care is inadequate, we can consider it due to waste and inefficiency of the bureaucracy, not due to our insufficient funding. Thirdly, it permits the carrying out of specific agendas as noted above.

In reality, there is both underfunding *and* inefficiency. We should expect the government to address the inefficiency. And, we should expect government and health care leaders—and we citizens—to address the level of financial support. Those at the very top of the bureaucracy who have power to set the policy and the tone—and to spend the dollars—must bear tremendous responsibility. They also have a tremendous opportunity.

. . .

You would not usually choose to have yourself or a family member cared for in a public facility. For one thing, the care is often by the least experienced or more marginal of practitioners. These are often training grounds for medical students and residents. Those in training love these facilities because they "get to do more." This translates as, "I get to learn because there are fewer skilled people who will do the work."

In addition to staff problems, there is also a pervasive inefficiency in management and treatment. The ACLU had helped institute a lawsuit aimed at Illinois' Department of Mental Health and Developmental Disabilities alleging an extremely substandard (more like "subhuman") level of care to the mentally ill. The legal document putting forth the details reads more like a horror story than an official document.

Patients who may already be demoralized enough from their illnesses, don't need the added burden of the poor system of care so often found in the public sector. These patients—and their families—should be able to focus on the physical or mental problem rather than on dealing with an often incompetent and uncaring bureaucracy.

And taxpayers, already feeling overburdened, don't wish to pay for both current waste and future expenses resulting from the consequences of poor care. Care for public sector patients could probably be less expensive if provided in the *private* sector, which is markedly more efficient. A favorite term used in the public sector is "deflected." In practical terms, this often translates as, "We got them off our backs by sending them somewhere else." Perhaps this "deflection" should be more often to private facilities rather than just back and forth between various public ones.

. . .

What's a person to do if they or a family member are receiving public sector care? First, generally try *not* to have this occur. If it does, be even more vigilant and alert than in the private sector. Work even harder implementing the "Four Steps to Better Care." If you're not being presented with diagnostic or treatment options which you know are available in the private sector, insist on knowing why. Just because services are free or at a reduced cost, doesn't mean patients shouldn't get reasonable care or can't ask for (and expect) understandable answers to appropriate questions.

Finally, be realistic. You will almost certainly have to lower your expectations, at least in terms of some of the attributes we expect of civilized health care. These include a reasonably pleasant setting, courtesy, and comfort. (Not that the private sector of the health care system is necessarily a paragon of these.)

And while the following is certainly not said to demean those who are working hard in the public interest, nevertheless, a bureaucratic official is *not* your physician and can't relate to you in the same healing fashion.

. . .

For as long as a two-tier system continues, it should at least be better than it is. Society needs to fund it adequately and its bureaucrats and staff should be held to greater accountability.

If we were ever to have a national system which provided everyone with equal access to quality care, a real problem would arise with regard to the fate of the public sector. With a greater access to first-tier care, how many of those now using the public sector would continue? A real stretch of one's optimism would be required to believe that the public sector could be brought up to such high standards that patients would want to stay with most of its facilities. Would public facilities just close their doors? We'd probably be better off if many of them did just that. But, for at least a while, this is neither likely nor desirable.

Even now, the public sector provides something of a window into the "soul" of government-controlled health care. Someday we may all be involved in what resembles a public sector system as our nation moves into a new era of health care delivery. But right now, be especially cautious if involved in the public sector. This system is often a "shame-on-us" as a supposedly caring society. We should be taking a very careful look at it—and at its possible alternatives.

CHAPTER 13

Mental Health Services and Stigma

Pearl:

If you see a psychiatrist, try to avoid being over-diagnosed and over-medicated.

The mentally ill are more like us than they are different from us. This is a great truth of life. I learned it from one of my wisest teachers while studying psychiatry. I would like to add my own corollary to it: Not only are they like us, they *are* us.

A related truth is this: No matter who you are, or how many advantages you have, at some point life will threaten to overwhelm you emotionally. A basic understanding of mental illness and the system which deals with it can be of great assistance when this crisis comes. To further understanding, I've divided the material in this chapter into the following two major areas: (1) exploring some of the uncertainties and confusing issues surrounding mental illness (such as "what is normal?" and stigma), and (2) providing some practical information for dealing with the mental health system, especially with regard to using medication.

Confused? Don't Be!

What is the purpose of mental health care? One might simply say that the purpose is to treat mental illness. But there are several problems with this approach. First, you must determine what is mental illness? Second, is mental illness on a psychological basis a significantly different entity than mental illness on a biological basis? (Psychiatrists sometimes uses the terms "biological," "organic," "clinical," and "physical" interchangeably.) And, what about distress that is a normal reaction to the realities of one's life? Is there a recognizable boundary at which such distress—such as grief over the loss of a loved one—crosses over to become a disorder?

The recognized medical specialty of psychiatry is difficult to define. You can choose from either of two following descriptions: (1) In *Psychiatry: Education and Image* (Brunner/Mazel, Inc.), psychiatry is referred to as "an unidentified technique applied to unspecified problems with unpredictable results." Or (2) —and this is what I tell my students—psychiatry is the study of the mind and how it adjusts both normally and abnormally; and if it adjusts abnormally, how that adjustment can be improved. If you don't like either of these definitions, then you must search further on your own—I've made my own uneasy peace with these.

It's difficult even to define what is normal. People have a wide range of acceptable behaviors which can differ markedly, especially from one cultural group to another. At various times in our lives, we all find important elements of our lives progressing for the better or the worse. Reacting to these elements in our own unique ways or being innately different to start with shouldn't necessarily indicate mental illness.

The essential point here is that what doesn't fall within the ill-defined boundaries of normal, by definition falls within the equally ill-defined boundaries of disorder. We use—or misuse—our labels for people fairly loosely, and almost certainly all of us fall into the "disorder" group at some time. One therapist might look at a patient's grieving as very normal; another may see it as quite pathological.

. . .

The distinction between biological illnesses and psychological illnesses is equally difficult to define. More and more, the emotional distresses of human beings are seen to have a biological basis. While I fully recognize the role of biology in our psychological lives, my personal feeling is that many mental health professionals have overreached the boundaries of our current knowledge as we tilt our explanations more to the biological side.

While psychiatrists talk about many patients having "chemical imbalances," it would be virtually impossible, in general, to demonstrate such an imbalance in patients by laboratory tests. (This comment excludes such physical problems as "low thyroid" which have mental symptoms.) In fact, patients might do well to note the response of their psychiatrists if challenged on this point. When told that, "You have a chemical imbalance," the patient might respond with, "I'd appreciate you running a test that would show this imbalance." My guess is that no test would be forthcoming. The fact that the 90's have been proclaimed "The Decade of the Brain" gives an indication of the current emphasis on the biological.

Patients will accept—and medical practitioners often feel more comfortable with—seeing things in a biological light. It's less stigmatizing to have one's depression caused by a "chemical imbalance" than by something deep within one's psyche. Biological causes put things more in the category of physical illnesses, such as appendicitis. That is, there is just a part that has gone wrong rather than a defect in what might be seen as the very essence of the individual.

A similar issue relates to psychiatric patients being told, "You have an illness like any other medical illness." Is it? I'm not trying to re-stigmatize mental illness. But I don't have a problem with admitting to having emotional distresses which *aren't* like a medical illness. Often these problems don't need medication. To lump so many mental illness together with diabetes and cancer is to do a disservice to those patients trying to fully *understand* what is happening to them psychologically.

In my clinical activities, I've prescribed psychiatric medications extensively. But I do think that drugs have definite limitations. If it were somehow possible to do a sort of global measurement of the overall risks and benefits of all drug treatments versus all psychotherapy treatments, my guess would be that psychotherapy would come out on top with fewer risks and more benefits. Of course, there would be some patients who would receive virtually no benefits unless they were given appropriate medication.

Concepts of drug addiction treatment are an especially murky area. This is another sphere where the mental health field seems to be moving more in the direction of organic causes and organic treatments. While research in such areas would be important, dogmatically applying any results prematurely would be a mistake. Still, this is an area where arguments could be made for any number of treatment approaches. Probably the single most important factor in a person's struggle against addiction is to take personal responsibility—at least of some level—for his/her own actions and life. I think various "programs" often have more to do with simply providing an opportunity to break one's destructive routine rather than providing any specific therapeutic benefit.

The issue of homelessness also impacts heavily within the mental health community. There's wide recognition that a high percentage of the homeless are mentally ill. Many have schizophrenia—an illness with a large biological component. At least part of the reason that we often avoid interaction with the homeless is that on some level we realize that we could be they. They are a visible reminder in our daily environment of our own vulnerabilities.

In truth, we know very little about the causes or boundaries of mental illness or how our treatments (either biological or psychotherapeutic) work. It's healthy to admit this lack of knowledge. Ultimately, an honest approach will be more productive in finding useful treatments as well as stimulating a more open dialogue between patient and therapist. In the meantime, we still need to understand each person as an *individual.*

. . .

I think that much of the stigma in psychiatry occurs when we conceptualize the illness as equivalent to the person, that the person is no longer the same person when he or she has a mental illness, but that the very "soul" has changed. (In fact, *psyche* comes from the Greek word for *soul.*) If I have appendicitis, my appendix is defective, but I am still me. But if I have manic-depression, I am a manic-depressive and perhaps it is I who am defective; my "soul" is broken.

People often feel more in control, more powerful, when they compare themselves to the mentally ill. In fact, it's a common experience on inpatient psychiatric units to hear patients say that they thought they were in bad shape until they saw the condition of other patients. "I'm not as bad off as I thought," they might say. I don't see this as necessarily a therapeutic response.

Maybe it's *necessary* for those who consider themselves healthy to be able to stigmatize the mentally ill. Perhaps it is a way of keeping "them" separate from "us." As long as they are stigmatized and apart from us, we may feel less vulnerable.

Certainly, there are other contributing causes to stigma, including concern over violence in the mentally ill and the fear of the unknown which permeates our "knowledge" of psychiatry.

. . .

With regard to therapists, it has been said that the best ones are those who are actually "sick" enough themselves to be able to understand what's happening to the patient, but healthy enough to be able to do something about it. I think there is an element of truth to this. Workers in the mental health field are often those who are struggling with their own distresses. To some extent they sort out these problems through their studies and their work with others. This may not be the healthiest of situations, but it seems to be the way it is. And, there are important insights therapists can gain from their own battles.

(Physicians—psychiatric and otherwise—don't wish to be seen as impaired any more than anyone else. So, because of their high profile, they may be especially reluctant to seek mental health services. To be caught doing so could wound their own self-image, or alter how patients and colleagues see them, or even jeopardize their professional licenses. Yet, doctors who are depressed, drinking to excess, or otherwise mentally compromised can be inefficient and unavailable at best or dangerous and deadly at worst.)

Whether they are ill or not, psychiatrists and other mental health professionals deal with much paradox, controversy, and uncertainty in their work. Perhaps one of the marks of an effective mental health practitioner is his or her ability to hold in mind opposing perspectives and not become paralyzed by these. While therapists explain, for example, that patients must do much of the work of therapy themselves, the therapists may hold themselves out as a major necessary ingredient for recovery.

. . .

Almost all patients can feel threatened by their illnesses, but the mentally ill are perhaps even more vulnerable to this. They may feel a greater loss of control and a greater sense of disintegration as human beings. This is probably more true of the chronically mentally ill, for example, those patients with schizophrenia. And, sometimes patients are so deeply affected that they don't even realize they are ill.

People should be aware that some psychiatric illnesses are fairly acute and are quite treatable: Once recognized, they are treated successfully, and fall into the background of a person's life. Even patients with more chronic problems can benefit to varying degrees by treatment.

Families often share in a sense of disintegration and loss of control. They had expectations. They made plans. They may see these expectations crumble in the face of sometimes unrelenting mental illness. This changes the family situation dramatically. Its members can feel powerless. Not only have they suffered a loss, they sometimes even feel in physical danger from their chronically ill family member.

On a larger plane, society might have even invented mental illness if it did not exist. Mental illness, to some extent, can play the role of the devils and gods of old. At least these ancient spirits provided previous cultures a way of understanding the incomprehensible. Today, if we perceive our God or our philosophy as being inadequate at providing order, we can turn to mental health professionals. (The kids aren't bad, they're just "ill.") If the professionals can provide a label and a treatment for a disorder, we feel we have some modicum of understanding and control over it. But in truth, in turning some problems over to professionals and throwing up our own hands, we have failed.

In spite of the limitations of the field, there is much that patients (non-physicians often see "clients") can be offered through mental health services. The next section will deal with some practical issues. A special focus in this chapter will be the use of medications. Psychotherapy was discussed in some detail in Chapter 8 in "Treatment."

Understanding and Using the System

Medications for mental illness are both over- and underused. There are many people suffering needlessly despite the availability of appropriate biological approaches. But at the same time, medications are also grossly overused. These excesses can roughly be put in three categories: First, there are patients who do not need to be treated with medication at all, but receive it anyway. Second, there are those who are treated with "endless psychopharmacology:" When one medicine doesn't work, it's on to the next, and the next, and the next. While there may be some validity to this progression, it should be a red flag for the patient to further discuss the matter with the practitioner. Third (and this is sometimes combined with endless psychopharmacology), is the prescribing of multiple medications at the same time. Here again, there can be some validity to this approach, but it also should be a warning signal for the patient to further question the clinician or to get a second opinion. To whatever extent possible, "less is more" in medication management.

The psychiatric medications which seem to live up to their image more than others are lithium and antipsychotics. When antidepressants work, they can be marvelous. But, often they fall far short of expectations. The use of anti-anxiety agents is more controversial than the other medications mentioned, but they certainly can have appropriate applications.

Virtually all medications have a risk. And psychiatric medications have some unique ones of their own. Much too often, practitioners see prescribed medications used by patients in suicide attempts. The treatment turns into a self-destructive weapon.

Also, prescribing a medication can give a message to the patient that the illness can't be dealt with in any other way. This can forestall the use of psychotherapy where it might otherwise have been helpful. (Keep in mind that from a physician's point of view, it's much easier to write a prescription than it is to see someone an hour a week for psychotherapy.) While in some cases, medications are prescribed to help with behavior that the patient can't control, in other cases drugs inappropriately give the message that "you're not responsible for your behavior—so the mental health system will assume responsibility."

Sometimes there is room for choice by patients regarding various medication approaches, or even a choice between psychotherapy or medications. The patient should be given the opportunity for as much involvement and selection as reasonable.

Mention should also be made here of electroconvulsive therapy. Most people generally think of this treatment as fairly brutal. It consists of providing an electric current to the brain, causing the person to have a convulsion. It's used primarily, but not exclusively, in the treatment of depression. For those problems for which it is indicated, it can be a superb treatment. Its image as inherently bad treatment is undeserved.

Mental health services can be very expensive. The cost can be looked at from two prospectives. First, relief of suffering due to mental illness can come at a cost far less than that of major surgeries and with just as much, if not more, benefit. On the other hand, many people receive services which are unnecessary or for which there are better alternatives. Inappropriate services are too costly at *any* price. In-patient adolescent services have been notoriously abused.

Alcoholism is one of those problems for which various approaches are available. Philosophically, I consider it less of a "disease" and more of a decision coming out of a troubled life. I want to emphasize that this is a purely personal opinion. In any given case, mental health practitioners may or may not do any better job than either A.A. or the individual who simply decides for himself or herself that it is time to put the bottle aside and get on with life. This isn't to say that a drinking problem may not be part of an overall psychological dysfunction by the patient which might need specific attention. Alcoholism is one of those very controversial areas—firm answers are hard to come by. Until such answers are available, I think that varied approaches and vigorous debate can both be justified.

. . .

Patients may find it helpful, perhaps even necessary, to develop their own philosophical approaches to both their care and their lives. These can serve as anchors in especially stormy times. A philosophical approach can help any of us, regardless of being "normal," physically ill, or mentally ill. Paradoxically, it may be very practical to be philosophical.

People with chronic mental illnesses which seem resistant

to treatment may need to search for valid philosophical reasons to aid them in not only enduring life, but even enjoying life. For them, the question may be, "How do I live with the unlivable?" There is an answer, but the search can be difficult.

Mental illness can also provide a valuable, if not painful, learning experience. People who have suffered severe emotional distress (or who have witnessed that of a loved one) can emerge from the process stronger and wiser. They can have a better understanding of themselves, as well as the struggles and imperfections of everyone else.

. . .

There are other specific practical approaches which a patient can use. Primary among these are using the "Four Steps to Better Care"—understanding, involvement, responsibility, authority. In Chapter Ten, I provided a generic list of questions for patients to address to virtually any practitioners. Here I will add a number of questions which can be additionally helpful in mental health settings, depending upon the circumstances:

- Why do you say that? (This can be used in response to virtually any explanation the practitioner puts forward.)
- What's the basis for that diagnosis?
- What's the basis for your treatment plan?
- Why medication?
- Why not medication?
- Why psychotherapy?
- Why not psychotherapy?
- Why both therapy and medication together?

Basically, the same material addressed in earlier chapters regarding interactions with doctors and hospitals applies here. In interacting with the mental health system, however, it may be especially valuable to keep your own records, as care can be particularly confusing. Since treatment alternatives can be so varied, it can be especially important for patients to have a willingness to explore options. This is also an area where family and friends may be able to play a greater role. Unfortunately, the nature of the illness may cause loved ones to be further isolated from the patient.

. . .

Finally, to conclude a discussion of practical aspects of mental illness, let's take a brief look at legal issues. Nowhere else within the health care field do clinical and legal issues intersect so routinely.

There is a vast body of law in this country which addresses various aspects of mental illness. Laws can vary greatly from state to state. Some of these issues are the rights of the mentally ill (including the right to own firearms), involuntary (forced) administration of medications, involuntary hospitalization, and interaction of the mentally ill with the criminal justice system.

An extremely important area of law is that regarding confidentiality. Confidentiality is one of the bulwarks upon which the relationship between patient and therapist is built. It can greatly enhance the cooperative effort between them. At the same time, it can further isolate families from information which they desire and which some people would argue should be made available to them. Also, confidentiality is not absolutely guaranteed, but might be broken for a variety of reasons such as involvement of the patient in child abuse or if the patient presents a serious danger to self or others.

The guiding principle to be applied to much of the above is the *individualization* of service. In mental health, it's not possible to use a "one size fits all" approach.

. . .

Mental health care is a paradox. On the one hand, it can offer remarkable relief from some emotional suffering; on the other hand, its arrogance, isolation from the real world, and over-reaching can also add significantly to the patients' distress. It's also perplexing; I realize that I haven't resolved all the issues I've raised. Practitioners should keep in mind that psychiatry is the least scientifically grounded of the medical specialties, but the one requiring the greatest "art." Meanwhile, patients must be particularly vigilant when obtaining mental health services. The additional obstacle of stigma further complicates the healing process.

While patients (and families, when appropriate) can do much to improve the level of care received by insisting on involvement, the major burden must be upon we professionals. We need to accept our limitations and ignorance, and arrogance should be put aside. Practitioners have many positive tools that are available to relieve patients' suffering. They should use them with skill, compassion—and restraint.

CHAPTER 14

Living With Chronic Illness

Pearl:
Remember, "chronic" means long, not devastating.

It's one thing to feel acutely miserable with the flu, a broken leg, or appendicitis. But at least we can anticipate that our suffering will end shortly. With chronic illness we have no such hope.

By definition, a chronic illness is *long*—although it doesn't necessarily last a lifetime. It can be, but isn't always, serious. For instance, I will die some day, having had acne virtually all my life, but it won't be the acne which will kill me. Chronic illnesses can be either physical or emotional in nature. Diabetes, multiple sclerosis, AIDS, emphysema, and schizophrenia are a few other examples of such problems. I also include injuries resulting in prolonged disability here.

The duration of a chronic illness sets it apart in three important ways. First, it provides the opportunity for ongoing patient education. Second, it frequently requires a significant change in lifestyle. Third, the patient will do better by developing a mindset of philosophical accommodation to any resulting disability. These aspects will be considered within the following discussion of psychological and practical factors.

. . .

Chronic illnesses can have tremendous emotional impact. People with serious chronic illnesses or disabilities face formidable tasks. They have suffered a loss of function and/or ability which they cannot ignore. Additionally, they must give priority to treatment or to the accommodation of limitations in their lives. They may have to give themselves injections of medication, schedule frequent doctors appointments or therapy sessions, or use a prosthetic device such as an artificial limb. There is a direct effect that these problems have on their lives, careers, and families. Also, there is the impact upon these patients of the reactions of others regarding their problem—pity, disgust, distancing, and so on.

People with chronic illnesses often share a number of characteristics. They may have a heightened awareness of the strength and frailties of the human mind and body. They usually have an acute awareness and understanding of the health care system with which they must interact. They recognize a sense of isolation, of being "different." They accept, or at least recognize, their limitations, while hopefully acknowledging their continuing capabilities.

Through all of this, they must reach an accommodation which will allow them to make peace with themselves, which will allow them to see their positive role in society (a society which often values strength and vigor above all else). Success in this task comes partially through a sense of commitment by the patient to focus on *ability*. Ideally, this is matched by support from the physician, other caregivers, family, friends, and work associates.

The emotional impact that a chronic illness can have on a family can be as dramatic as its impact on the patient. The family will participate in the patient's loss and suffering. Not only can the family's *lifestyle* change, but sometimes their *lives* will change as well.

. . .

There are practical steps that those with chronic illnesses can take to ease their burden and suffering. One of the most important aspects of having a chronic illness is to have as much clinical knowledge about it as possible. This kind of knowledge can help patients to deal with the illness more effectively as well as work more intelligently with their physicians and other caregivers. Informed patients can more fully understand the purposes of various recommendations, understand the caregivers' discussions and instructions more fully, and be better prepared to ask important questions.

A crucial piece of information which the patient should have is an understanding of the course of the illness. Will it be filled with remissions and exacerbations (an up-and-down course)? Is the course basically a stable one? Is it one of progressive deterioration, or is it terminal? What sort of additional problems and complications can be anticipated along the way? All of this information will help the patients to cope with their illnesses more competently as well as to plan their lives more effectively.

If you are chronically ill, read as much as you can about your ailment. Many books have been written regarding specific illnesses, such as hypertension, diabetes, schizophrenia, depression, and more. Also consider joining support groups or national associations which deal with your particular problem. If you have on-line access, use your computer to search for information.

If your physician is not particularly expert in your area of illness, your own personal education may be even more important. It often happens that patients wind up knowing more about their illnesses than their physicians. Then, patients can (gently and with tact) provide to their doctors material which they have found helpful.

An alternative approach is to have one's ongoing care under the direction of a specialist in that particular field. If this isn't possible, an occasional consultation with such a specialist can aid the physician who is working directly with the patient on a regular basis. Whether you are working with a specialist or not, it can be helpful to have routinely scheduled visits and testing, rather than just a "call if there are any problems" arrangement. For instance, the patient and physician might work out a program where routine appointments occur every month or three months or six months. Various laboratory test might be done between some of these appointments, with the results being communicated to the patient.

During all of this, it's especially important for a patient to keep his or her own set of medical records. Ideally, this would include copies of discharge summaries, consultation reports, test results, and surgical reports. Because the illness is chronic and by its nature lasts a long time, a patient may go through many physicians. A good set of records will be of great benefit as the patient encounters new caregivers. A separate diary, which patients can develop themselves, can help chart the ups and downs of their illness as changes occur with various treatments and events in their lives.

Because of the disruptive effects that chronic illnesses can have on lives, sticking to appropriate personal routines can become particularly important. Illnesses are innately chaotic already, so if you find yourself in this situation, keep your life as normal as possible. Regardless of the nature of the illness or incapacity, allow time in your life for recreation, family, travel, and whatever pleasures your illness and finances will allow. The travel industry is becoming much more user-friendly these days for people with disabilities.

Work routines can often be maintained. Many people with chronic illnesses continue to be productive employees or can even become entrepreneurs The Americans with Disabilities Act may help with employment issues.

The impact of a chronic illness upon the family can be as great as it is on the patient. The family may be dealing with resultant financial responsibilities, disruption of future plans, changes in current activities, fear of anticipated loss, or even anxiety and guilt.

In families where a member has a chronic illness, good communications are especially important. The patient will usually be painfully aware of the ramifications of the illness. Feelings and concerns should be shared as much as possible.

I recently read of the existence of a support group for spouses of the chronically ill. Overall, this sounds like a great idea. But, in the process of seeking their own support, family members should take care not to make the patient feel worse for being the source of "the problem."

Family members can grow even stronger and more mature by their involvement with an ill member. While they might not see the situation as a blessing, they could come to understand their role as one of the finest expressions of a civilized society—caring for others.

As always, be aware of the "Four Steps to Better Care." Because of the opportunity for studying the clinical condition during the prolonged course of a chronic illness, there is a greater possibility of more understanding and active involvement. Since caregivers sometimes turn away from those with long-term illnesses, feeling that no "cure" is in sight, such patients may have to be even more self-reliant.

. . .

Life can be tough enough without the constant additional burden of a chronic illness. But with a reasonable approach, the situation doesn't always have to be a major obstacle.

The keys to success are: obtaining education about the illness; having access to quality care; accommodating but limiting any changes in lifestyle; developing a productive philosophical mindset; and *carrying on* while focusing on one's strengths and abilities, not one's disabilities.

CHAPTER 15

Undiagnosable Conditions

Pearl:

Don't be overly impressed by a "diagnosis;" it may be nothing more than a sophisticated expression of a doctor's ignorance.

As I write this chapter, I am awaiting my own test results from a sonogram examination which uses the reflection of sound waves to provide pictures of the inside of the body. My first worry is that it will show a serious illness such as cancer. My second worry is that it won't show any disease at all. Because if the test reveals nothing, what would I "do" with the pain and discomfort I have been suffering?

This kind of situation—symptoms, but no objective findings—is common. Examples could include back pain, headache, tiredness, or depression. Regardless of the specific complaint, the result is a serious conundrum for both patient and physician.

There are a number of possibilities facing anyone in this situation: Has the diagnosis been missed? Does it have more to do with body *function* (which may be more difficult to detect) rather than body *structure*? Is the problem too small (or "too early") to be picked up? Is it psychological? Will people think the patient is faking? Few of these choices are good.

The situation faced by a physician treating such a patient is also less than ideal. He or she may have to deal with (1) a symptom pattern ("history") which doesn't neatly fit any illness known to that particular doctor and/or (2) no helpful objective findings on physical examination or testing, i.e., nothing that can be demonstrated.

Faced with this situation, the physician might:

1. Say "I don't know."
2. Give the problem a psychiatric label.
3. Take a more-or-less educated guess so as to come up with a medical label.

Of course, the doctor could also discuss the possibility of ordering tests, referring the patient to another physician, or simply following his or her progress over time while deferring the diagnosis.

Only if the physician admits that it is not possible to come up with a diagnosis at that time could the problem be considered potentially *un*diagnosable. If an inappropriate psychiatric or medical label is applied, it can be considered as *mis*diagnosed. An undiagnosable problem is rarely left with that particular label for very long as it is frequently followed by a misdiagnosis which can be tragic for the patient. You're better off being undiagnosed. At least then, there's still an open question rather than a closed mistake.

Misdiagnoses can arise because the medical profession is not as sharp at diagnosing as it advertises itself to be. Physicians are uncomfortable with their ignorance and tend to deny their limitations. When they don't know something, they're inclined to convince themselves, and the patient, that their hunch is the same as reality. Rarely will they say, "I'll look it up."

Doctors aren't the only ones who are uncomfortable with the idea of listing in a medical record that there is "no diagnosis" or that the diagnosis is "deferred": Patients often don't like these designations either. They want a concrete label to link to their distress. So do insurance companies. In addition, medical administration abhors a missing diagnosis. A diagnosis—even a wrong one—is what's wanted. The doctor usually obliges.

. . .

Issues surrounding the diagnostic process are somewhat complex. First, let's trace the development of the situation: Patient sees doctor. Doctor listens to and examines patient. The diagnosis is not clear-cut—it could be almost anything. Even testing, sometimes with "false-negative" or "false-positive" results, doesn't always help.

The doctor makes his or her best guess, but *records* it as if it's a certainty. Almost as soon as the misdiagnosis is made, it's as if it was carved in granite. A treatment is prescribed based on the erroneous label. The patient fails to improve. Like a dog chasing its tail, round after round of inappropriate treatments chasing after inaccurate diagnoses can occur.

The patient faces two more problems in addition to the misdiagnosis itself. First is that he or she may fail to improve. I say "may" because even with misdiagnosis, the symptoms might improve for a number of reasons: A treatment picked for the wrong reason might be effective because medications can have a broad spectrum of effects and fortuitously hit the target anyway; or there may be a placebo effect; the disease may simply run its course and the patient will recover; or—in the worst-case scenario—the symptoms are merely "masked" with a temporary improvement as the disease progresses, sometimes to a fatal outcome.

The second problem the patient can face is additional distress due to anxiety, uncertainty, self-doubt, and even from a sense of isolation. It's harder to share one's suffering when that suffering is so hard to pin down. Lack of progress raises the issue of, "Is it me?" And a lingering (but often unspoken) question of, "Is it the doctor?" adds to the problem.

If there isn't a mental illness causing the symptoms, one may very well develop as the patient struggles with the problem. Then the picture can really become murky: An improperly recognized physical illness in a person who now also has emotional symptoms. As in *Alice's Adventures in Wonderland*, things get "curiouser and curiouser!"

Medicine is still more of an art than a science—and today's doctors often aren't very good artists. Technology is their god. The history (information gathered from the patient) should still routinely be more important than tests or even physical examination. But taking a good history requires time. And doctors—caught up in technology and being cost-effective—have less and less time for listening.

Patients can unintentionally complicate the history either because of inadequate recall of the symptoms and timing or because they have a difficult time "reading" their own bodies. The location of a pain in the abdomen may be very ill-defined, yet we try to say that it's "right here." The doctor may even encourage this, saying, "Point to the pain with one finger." The more experienced I become as a physician, the more impressed I am with how hard it really is to pinpoint the location of a discomfort.

Unfortunately, our scientific tools for diagnosis are still in their infancy. They're crude—often operating at about the same level of accuracy as trying to examine and describe Da Vinci's "Last Supper" from 100 feet away. Maybe all we can tell from that distance is that "it's a bunch of people sitting at a table."

Too, there are a number of diagnoses and conditions which are problematic for either the physician or the patient. These include such diverse entities as chronic fatigue syndrome, fibromyalgia, premenstrual syndrome (PMS), environmental illness, hypoglycemia, irritable bowel syndrome, and Lyme disease.

More in the purview of psychiatrists are posttraumatic stress disorder (PTSD), multiple personality disorder (recently renamed "dissociative identity disorder"), some diagnoses of "depression," attention-deficit/hyperactivity disorder (ADHD), some addictions, false memory syndrome, and others.

Many of the above problems are very confusing issues. They may have multiple or perplexing symptoms or even be of questionably diagnostic validity. I won't even try to present the controversies, much less lay out specific plans for dealing with each. The point to be made here is simply that these and other labels can seriously confound the diagnostic and treatment process.

Patients and physicians should always be open to the possibility of error in almost any diagnosis, but especially if treatment proves unsuccessful or if the implications of the diagnosis are particularly critical for survival. I like to think of such an approach as healthy skepticism in the service of better care.

Finally, women should be more skeptical of diagnoses. Simply having more major organs and a more complex physiology puts women at risk for having more diagnoses and more surgeries. Couple this with the medical profession's male dominance and ignorance of female psychology, and you have the perfect setting for diagnostic dilemmas.

. . .

What can you do if you feel your condition is undiagnosable or that it has been misdiagnosed?

First, try to assist the physician as much as possible. Note your symptoms carefully as they develop, perhaps using a diary format. Then be prepared to summarize the difficulty as succinctly as possible. Follow the "Four Steps to Better Care."

Physicians do have ways of productively addressing difficult diagnostic cases. I give my students a list of several approaches to use. These include being honest but supportive with the patient

("I don't know what this is, but we can work on it together"), and being a good manager in coordinating all efforts to reach a diagnosis, including gathering old records and requesting new consultations.

If you feel that the case has gone beyond the efforts of your doctor, what's next? Worth considering is an appointment at one of our nation's major diagnostic centers. Many people turn to such facilities as Mayo Clinic, Cleveland Clinic, Johns Hopkins, Carle Clinic, and many others. Or, if your doctor hasn't suggested a more local consultation, you can always ask for one. Of course, you can always try another physician without a referral from your own doctor. "Free-lancing" to other care on your own can have an up-side and a down-side. The advantage of free-lancing is that you not only get another exam, but one with a new perspective without any bias from, or possible obligation to, a referring physician. The disadvantages, however, are numerous: Your selection can turn out to be a poor choice; some tests may be unnecessarily repeated; findings may not get communicated back to someone who will work with you on a more regular basis; your health plan may not pay for this exam; or you may be embarking on a whole series of unproductive "doctor hopping" experiences.

If physicians need to use good judgment, so do patients. Don't let desperation overshadow yours.

. . .

If you have an undiagnosable illness, the accompanying chart (Figure 2) may help you locate where you sit in this uncomfortable situation.

At the far left hand corner of the page, note that there are some diagnoses which simply can't be made. They are undiagnosable either because of the limited progression of the illness or because of the limitations of our current technology. With the passage of time or with the development of new technology, the nature of the undiagnosable illness may become quite clear.

The next heading of "Tough Cases" represents challenges to even a competent diagnostician. Even so, the diagnosis can be made with the exercise of finely honed expertise or extra effort. Sometimes, additional or more sophisticated testing can help. Symptoms which occur intermittently rather than constantly often fall into this category.

Many illnesses are relatively diagnosable, tricky but still discernible. However, even these can be misdiagnosed by physicians who rush to conclusions. A too "cost-effective" health care plan can be a contributory factor.

Even with proper diagnosis, as the chart shows, the patient may not improve. This can be due to a number of reasons: right diagnosis, but wrong treatment; "proper" treatment, but lack of response to initial appropriate efforts; or non-compliance by the patient in following the physician's recommendations.

Of course, even the diagnosis doesn't always matter. Thanks to the marvelous healing power of the mind and body, we sometimes get better either without, or in spite of, care. Just being aware of the possibilities in this overall scheme can help patients to more intelligently consider their options.

Whether the problem is truly undiagnosable or misdiagnosed, a certain philosophical acceptance may be in order: "I'll continue on with my life the best I can while solving this problem." The additional suffering caused by an undiagnosable or misdiagnosed problem can be greater than the suffering with some diagnosed illnesses that are even quite serious. If the additional suffering is adversely affecting your life, you can seek out the services of a mental health professional to help you through this difficult period.

If you're doing all you can, but still aren't improving, perhaps your doctor isn't providing either enough time or expertise. Consider the options presented in the discussion in Chapter 18, "Dissatisfaction with Care."

A final note on an important practical consideration: Don't forget that any of us could currently have a serious illness without

Diagnostic and Outcome Possibilities Flow Chart
Figure 2

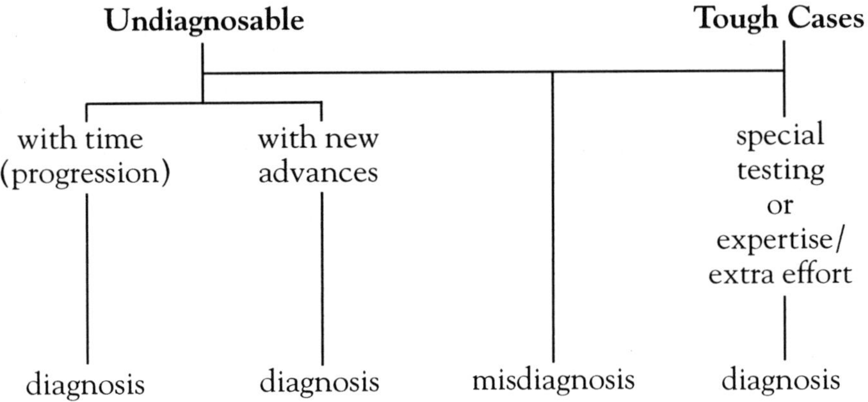

Note: The chart represents *some* of the possibilities, given here as examples only.

Figure 2 (continued)

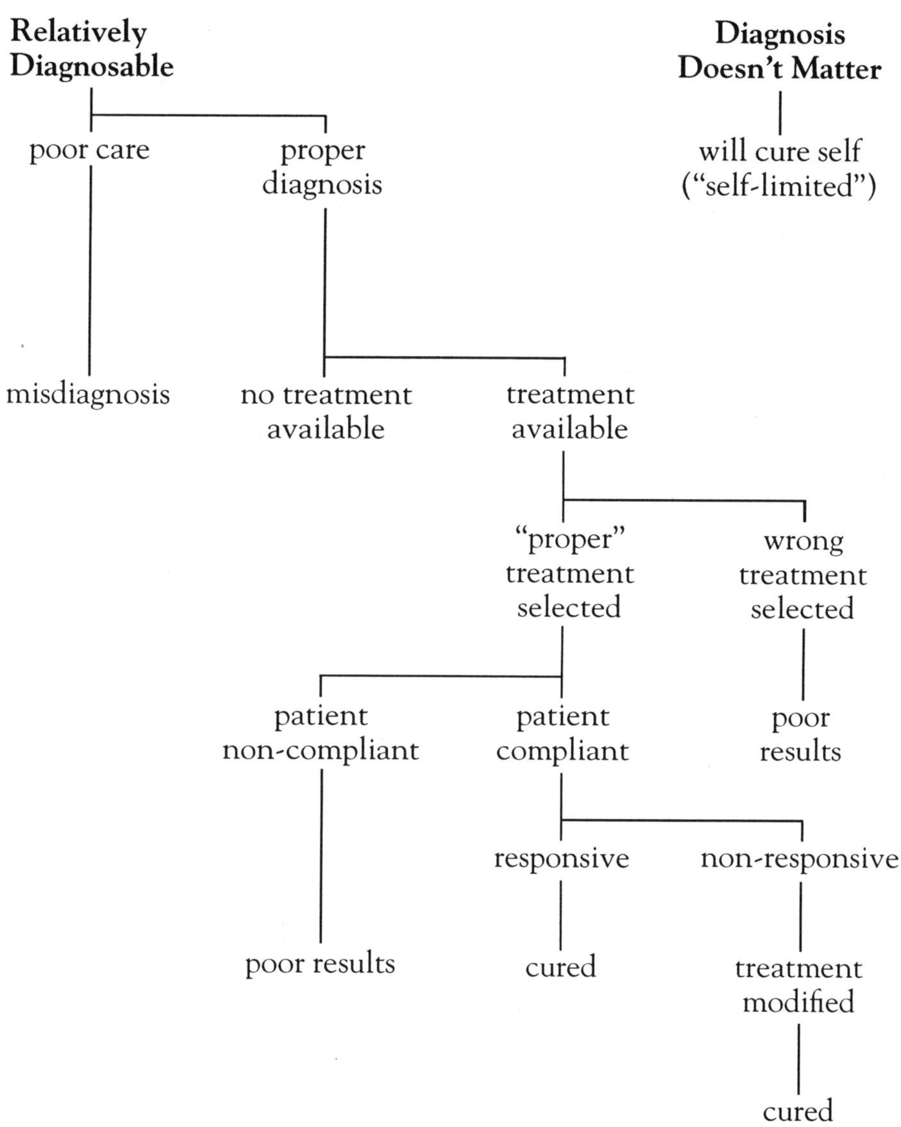

noticeable symptoms. Because we could become undiagnosable or be misdiagnosed at any time, we should all work out a lifetime plan of prevention *and* early detection. Work with your primary care physician. If there is a major role for family practitioners, this would be it!

. . .

The physician may ultimately come up with the answer to the problem, especially with the patient's help. ("When all else fails, ask the patient.") But this is a situation where patients may have to virtually become their own best resource—or risk years of chaos or disability.

If there's a short answer to the problem of having a difficult-to-diagnosis condition, it's this: Have a plan, be open to all possibilities (including physical or emotional), work with the best physician(s) you can find, persevere, and have a positive philosophical outlook until the problem is resolved. Such an outlook will be especially important if a problem is never resolved. Some aren't.

The diagnosis may eventually come with time, rather than be a "timely diagnosis." Hopefully, it will at least come in time for effective medical intervention.

CHAPTER 16

"Bad" Patients

Pearl:

Patients' care can be more affected by their attitudes than by their diagnoses.

In the sometimes convoluted thinking of health care, bad is good and good is bad.

If a patient wishes to be actively involved in his or her care and is appropriately inquisitive, probing, concerned, questioning, and not easily put off by inadequate answers from doctors or other providers, you might be tempted to think of him or her as a "good" patient. But you'd be wrong. Caregivers often see such people as nuisances—"bad" patients. I like to think of such people a "Type A-Positive" bad patients. "Type A" is for assertive, active, and alert; the "Positive" is because I think their stance is preferable.

But in defense of caregivers, there is another group: "Type O-Negative" bad patients. The "O" stands for obnoxious and obstructive. The "Negative" means these patients do more harm than good to themselves and to those they relate to (other patients, caregivers, and so on). They are correctly perceived as "bad," because that's what they are.

It's a common experience that the manner in which one person approaches another actually influences the response of the other person. Patients *and* doctors sometimes forget this. The results can be decreased effectiveness in a relationship which should have as much going for it as possible.

An ideal situation would be if sick and/or worried patients could always approach their physicians in the most efficacious manner and that physicians would respond in kind. Unfortunately, a patient's suffering often precludes this. They might try their best, but what comes out may sound argumentative, disrespectful, or even threatening. The caregiver can be immediately put off.

During their training, physicians should acquire an immunity to patients' communicative and emotional failures. Furthermore, doctors should learn ways to facilitate better communications. Some do. Many don't. It is the physician's responsibility to take the higher ground even when the patient is unable to do so.

The solution for helping physicians to work more effectively with patients begins with a more careful selection of medical students. It continues with training that shows how to develop good communications and relationships (both types of which are currently minimally provided, if at all). And it culminates in learning at the bedside from excellent role models.

For patients, the solution lies in doing their best during difficult situations. Having your act together during some of life's non-medical learning experiences provides good practice. Having a plan and being properly prepared—as this book has been urging—also helps.

. . .

In this chapter, the focus will be on patients. Patients bring all their old "baggage" and their psychological make-up into the clinical setting. Life's disappointments, frustrations, joys, and successes come right in with them, shaping any new encounters and experiences.

Additionally, the circumstances of the ailment can magnify the patient's suffering, anxiety, and uncertainty. Lack of income or insurance can put the patient more on the defensive by increasing fears of abandonment or inadequate care. The clinical setting also adds its own special stresses to patient behavior. Being in unfamiliar and frightening surroundings without the usual supports worsens the situation.

The amount of psychological baggage a patient brings into the patient-doctor relationship has an impact. Those who are relatively unencumbered are more likely to be Type A-Positive—assertive, active, and alert.

If the baggage is too great or the communication skill is too poor, people can come across as obnoxious and obstructive. These latter are the Type O-Negative patients.

Since physicians have gotten their share of criticism in this book, a few words devoted to bawling out patients would seem in order. There *are* a fair number of Type O-Negative patients whose attitudes are really bad. And they aren't doing themselves any favors. In addition to being obnoxious and obstructive, they have a number of other unproductive behaviors. They may expect too much from their care. They may jump haphazardly from doctor to doctor in search of relief, which remains elusive. And, once involved with a caregiver, they may treat him or her more as an adversary than as a partner. Such patients often are not very informed about either their own history or their illness. They frequently aren't prepared to appropriately use whatever appointment time is available.

These patients may want to be diagnosed over the phone and may demand an accompanying prescription. They often prefer to dictate their own care without having a good foundation for doing so. When inpatient care is needed, they take a "hospital-as-hotel" approach. Staff are seen as their personal employees and are often treated without the simplest common courtesy.

When being seen as outpatients, the Type O-Negative patients can be extremely frustrating for physicians. They may wait until the end of an appointment to bring up additional problems which were not mentioned at either the time of scheduling or at the beginning of the interview. Their attitude can be seen as, "I've got a problem; now, what are you going to do about it?"

Obviously, these behaviors can result in some very adverse consequences. At a minimum, these patients seem to rub everyone the wrong way. People distance themselves from them. The patients are certainly not helping those trying to provide care.

Patients who are Type O-Negative—and even those who are already doing well as Type A-Positives—can all learn to do better. All patients can start by picking the right doctor. Not every physician is the right match for every patient, as personalities can clash. Some patients would do better in multi-specialty practice settings where consultants and primary care physicians work together in teams and where practice "coverage" can be more readily available. Patients can limit visits to the local "doc-in-a-box" if an ongoing physician-patient relationship is important to them (it ought to be).

Patients should also be realistic and have an awareness of the clinical limitations of caregivers to relieve suffering. Practitioners may feel practical constraints such as pressures to limit referrals or to limit appointment length in HMO settings. These can be serious problems of managed care.

It can be helpful for patients to channel some of their energies into self-help. Taking good general care of one's self, following prescribed medical programs responsibly, and being well-educated in health care matters are all reasonable approaches.

Being a Type A-Positive patient means utilizing the "Four Steps to Better Care." By now you will know these well:

understanding, involvement, responsibility, and authority. These can be used assertively but graciously, with appropriate questions based on common sense and one's personal research about a problem.

For the dyed-in-the-wool Type O-Negative patient, there is hope. These people can become aware of how they are perceived by others. They can at least practice minimal common courtesy ("please" and "thank you"). These patients can become well-informed. They may have to be ready to do as much as possible for themselves because caregivers may not provide the level of assistance desired or needed. Enlisting the participation of Type A-Positive family members or friends in the medical encounter, when practical and appropriate, can also help blunt some of the Type O-Negative patient's undesirable characteristics.

. . .

Type A-Positive patients will ultimately stand a better chance of receiving more productive care. They may initially, however, have some rough sledding as they find and "train" the right doctor for themselves. Their search may be more prolonged and their patience may be put to the test early on.

As health care delivery continues to change—and it surely will—patients will need all the advantages they can get in dealing with an increasingly impersonal and cost-conscious clinical environment. So, be a Type A-Positive if possible—and do it as well as you can. Or learn to be at least a tolerable Type O-Negative. Be as much of a productive force in your care as possible.

CHAPTER 17

Emergencies

Pearl:
If in doubt, assume you're having an emergency and respond accordingly.

A medical emergency presents the patient with a *double* dilemma: First, a crises of either the body or the mind, and second, a more subtle crisis of decision-making. Even if the emergency is potentially life-threatening in itself, it's the decision-making which can mean the difference between life and death.

In other words, what you or your family decide, and what your doctors decide, can have more serious consequences than what's wrong with you in the first place—even in very critical situations.

By making the wrong choice when options are available, defeat can be readily snatched from the jaws of victory. For example, a patient experiencing a heart attack may choose to delay an emergency room visit long after chest pains begin, or the ER staff may decide on a course of observation after a traumatic injury when a more aggressive treatment is indicated.

There are some simple ways you can tilt the wise-decision-making odds in your favor. Understand as much as you can about health problems in general. Be especially familiar with the emergencies which may arise from your own known health problems. Be knowledgeable about the resources and reputations of practitioners and facilities in your area.

Make as many decisions as possible in advance of the emergency. When the emergency occurs, it may already be too late for much productive decision-making. In other words, be prepared so that you can largely switch your brain to "automatic" when the crisis begins. Pilots are like this. They don't try to figure out anew how to respond to each emergency situation aboard their aircraft. They have studied and rehearsed the most likely situations time and time again. They already have a plan. So should you.

. . .

Our sense of vulnerability increases at the time of an emergency. We are aware that something is happening to us *now*. And we are generally aware of its implications for our survival.

The crisis is largely unpredictable. And it is a relatively unique situation within most people's experiences, so most aren't likely to be ready to respond with maximum efficiency. There may be little time for careful, reflective thinking. Anxiety may cloud our deliberations. Choices may be limited. The situation may even be taken out of the individual's control by an ambulance crew, emergency room staff, or family. All of a person's life can suddenly be funneled down into one brief, chaotic episode. We become aware that resolution one way or another is likely to occur over the next few hours—or even sooner.

Your anxiety may be become your worst enemy at a time like this, blocking productive thinking and putting you at a disadvantage. Again, an aviation analogy is in order. Pilots need to remain calm during an emergency so that the enemy remains the emergency, not their own emotions. The same should be true for people experiencing a health crisis.

Fortunately, ER personnel are usually able to remain calm. First, the situation which is unique to you is likely to be commonplace to them. Secondly, it's not their lives—a circumstance which can be either good or bad. Of course, ER staffs are not totally immune to becoming unproductively anxious; but, as in other aspects of life, a little appropriate anxiety can be useful.

I think it is a myth that doctors have this driving force to "cheat death" in an emergency. What they have is a job to do. As professionals, they desire to do it well on the behalf of the patient. And they desire to do it well on their own behalf—to not screw up, look bad, or get sued.

. . .

How do emergency rooms really function? These facilities are generally seen as havens of refuge for those in critical medical need. But, all emergency rooms are not created equal. Some are well-equipped Trauma Centers, ready to receive those with severe, multiple injuries. Some don't even have a doctor present at all times. Visits to the emergency room of a small rural hospital can be much different, for better or for worse, than to one at "Mega-Center General."

Upon arrival, patients are generally "triaged," that is, prioritized by the staff in terms of appropriate order in which services will be provided to them. Consequently, there can be long waits for those not near the top of the more serious list. In extremely dire situations involving massive casualties, the very worst patients—those likely to die no matter what is done—will be passed over for care in favor of those with more of a chance to live.

If the emergency room has *any* doctor on the premises, the personnel will still probably need to call in a specialist (such as a neurosurgeon or cardiologist) when certain kinds of expertise are required. For this purpose, emergency rooms maintain "on-call" lists. Staff physicians generally take turns providing coverage on this schedule. Some doctors take this responsibility seriously and respond rapidly. Others can be slow to arrive, or even argue with the ER crew when their assistance is requested. At any rate, you may or may not be able to choose a specific doctor by name when you visit an ER.

There is a deliberateness within the hurried pace of an emergency room which patients and family often perceive as inaction. However, if diagnosis and treatment is to be properly carried out, this methodical approach is necessary. If things seem to be moving too slowly, patient and family should make inquiries in a non-threatening fashion, with increasing assertiveness as the situation may warrant.

Throughout all this, the inevitable paperwork of health care seeps in. It's helpful to have a family member to assist in providing some of the administrative information. Keeping a copy of your "Brief Personal Medical History Form" (Appendix B) in your car and/or on your person can be helpful at a time like this.

. . .

What are some of the additional practical aspects of a trip to the emergency room? Primary among these is to have a plan. It's helpful if you've considered in advance what facility you would like to use for emergency care and know whether or not you have a physician on the staff at that hospital. Having developed a personal set of guidelines for what you consider acceptable in the area of health care is also helpful.

Consider these questions in advance. Would you rather have your condition only stabilized so that you can be transferred to another facility and/or to physicians you know? Would you agree to heroic but possibly very damaging procedures that may result in your death or a severe disability? Would you insist on a second opinion prior to agreeing to any surgery? What if you're told that there's "no time" for a consultation? Is care by a family practitioner as acceptable to you as specialty care? When your initial plan fails, do you have a "plan B" ready for backup?

Additional concrete planning can be done in a number of areas. You can already have completed an "advance directive" as discussed earlier. Being familiar with your medical coverage and having your insurance card with you can be of great assistance. A MedicAlert bracelet can provide information about your allergies or serious illnesses. You can have a good grasp of your own history and be prepared to reiterate it quickly, giving only essentials.

Simply knowing how to present medical information to physicians can be a marked advantage. Much of this can be practiced during routine office visits. Stick to these essentials in emergency situations:

- What happened to you to put you in the emergency room?
- What are you experiencing in terms of symptoms?
- What operations and serious illnesses have you had?
- What medications do you take?
- What allergies do you have?

The ER staff is likely to ask you about all or most of these issues. Each point can provide critical information. All responses should be as brief as possible but as comprehensive as needed.

There are some buzz words that get a staff's attention more than others. Among these are "chest pain," "about to deliver," "suicidal," "bleeding," and "convulsed." However, even more impressive to staff than what you tell them is what they can see in terms of objective evidence. This would include things like being able to see external evidence of the injuries, blood coming out of any orifice, a fever registered on a thermometer, an abnormal EKG, or positive results from laboratory tests or X-rays.

As in other medical situations, the absence of hard clinical evidence can be detrimental to the patient. If you are really seriously in trouble, something will usually show up to provide documentation. If it doesn't, you're back to some of the issues already discussed in Chapter 15 on "undiagnosable conditions," and caregivers may quickly lose interest in your case. If this occurs in a potential emergency situation, you may have to ask for another opinion or request transfer directly to another facility. Neither of these are easily accomplished.

An emergency room may not wish to deal with a patient for a number of other reasons. It may not feel equipped to do so due to lack of special resources, or its hospital beds may already be filled to capacity. It may see the patient as undesirable due to lack of financial resources—or due to just plain obnoxiousness. Occasionally these patients are transferred to other facilities (a common experience for mental health patients). Depending on the hospital's motivation, this could represent a "dump."

If time and the nature of the emergency permits, bring whatever you can that may be useful for a possible hospital stay. If you have been keeping your own set of medical records at home, bring these, too. But there is a certain risk that caregivers may see your preparation in a less than positive light. When emergency room physicians see luggage at the side of the patient's gurney, they may sarcastically refer to it as a "positive suitcase sign," implying that this patient will be hard to get rid of. And ER staffs sometimes see the avoidance of admission as one of their prime tasks.

. . .

You may have to be your own best manager during an emergency room visit. Part of this effort would certainly involve utilizing the "Four Steps to Better Care." Doing so may be especially difficult under the circumstances, but it may also be especially important. To whatever extent possible, note people's names, titles, and faces. Try to keep a mental record of the proceedings. Ask for information as people interview you or come to you for information, specimens, or tests.

There are some things you don't want to do. If the visit isn't going well, try not to come across as too threatening, aggressive, obnoxious, disrespectful, or impatient. Do make your wishes or needs known, but do so in an appropriate manner. Family members can sometimes provide literally living-saving backup to you in this situation.

If you are dissatisfied with your caregiver or wish a second opinion on general principles, do whatever is reasonable to be seen by the type of physician you prefer. Ultimately, you can always at least ask for transfer or simply say "no" to recommendations. In rare situations, however, the emergency room staff may have the power to override any of your requests or preferences depending upon how critical your situation is. Hopefully, they will use their power with discretion and at the same time realize that the potential loss of control is part of patients' fears in visiting an emergency room.

. . .

Most emergency room visits do end with a discharge to home, not a disaster. The staff will probably give you some written information as you are preparing to depart. Regardless of what is on the paper, be sure that you talk to someone (ideally, the doctor who examined you) about your diagnosis and its significance. Know what you are suppose to do in terms of care at home. Have information regarding the purpose, interactions, and side effects of any medication which might be prescribed. If there is to be an outpatient follow-up visit, be sure you understand why, where, when, and with whom. And, especially understand what to do if your situation deteriorates or does not resolve itself as a result of any treatment or instructions given to you.

. . .

There are two tricks to better emergency care. First, simple preparation and forethought may be as important as your actual care in the ER. Second, at a time when the dramatic setting, hurried attitude of the staff, and your unfamiliarity with the situation may all encourage your passivity, this is when your involvement (or that of your family)—and the rest of the "Four Steps To Better Care"—can be especially important.

CHAPTER 18

Dissatisfaction With Care

Pearl:
The best tool for resolving dissatisfaction is often honest, open communication.

(*I Can't Get No) Satisfaction* is a song familiar to fans of the "Rolling Stones." But more and more, patients are singing the same refrain about their medical care. It's getting to be one of those tunes they can't seem to get out of their heads.

What is dissatisfaction? It could be described as a sense that (1) for some reason, clinical care is not being provided as it should be, (2) some other aspect of the patient-doctor relationship has gone awry, or (3) that something is seriously amiss within the delivery system—for example, you are being overcharged.

Who gets dissatisfied? Doctors can become dissatisfied in relationships with patients they would rather not see walk through the door at all. But the primary focus of this chapter will be from the patient's perspective.

What causes dissatisfaction? Sometimes it's stimulated by the unanticipated course of an illness. The patient expected to be doing better or to be cured, but, as time goes on, the results do not meet the expectations.

It could be that the patient's or family's expectations were unrealistic. Indeed, progress or relief may be occurring at the best possible rate. If this is the case, the physician may have been overly encouraging, or may not have clearly explained to the patient and family the likely course of the illness. Good communications are vital to a patient's satisfaction.

Without good communication, the seeds of dissatisfaction may be planted early. Ideally, the physician explains to the patient the recommendations and rationale behind a treatment program. The risks, benefits, and potential options should also be discussed. This is put in the context of what is generally expected (but not guaranteed) for the treatment of such a problem. (Mr. Jones, the medicine helps the majority of people like you, but not everyone.") The doctor should have a sense that the patient has a good understanding, has been given an opportunity to ask questions and, ultimately, has given an informed consent.

Was any room allowed for negotiation and compromise in this scenario? The physician may feel that more than just a single approach could be justified, and may be willing to select from among the alternatives the one with which the patient is most comfortable. However, physicians should not be put in the position of carrying out treatment with which they are in disagreement. If the physician disagrees with what the patient wants, it might be time to see what another physician thinks—for the sake of both parties.

A special case involving dissatisfaction occurs when the patient is forced into a relationship and/or treatment without any choice. This occurs often in mental health settings when patients in need of medication or hospitalization disagree with recommendations but are nevertheless legally forced to submit. This puts an additional burden upon the physician to try to develop the most positive relationship possible under the circumstances. Choices can be less dramatically limited in situations such as when the patient belongs to an HMO, lives in a small town, or goes to a public sector facility for financial reasons.

Assuming that there was a clear understanding and mutual cooperation, what else can cause dissatisfaction? Clinically poor or incompetent care is always a possibility. The fact that this happens far too often is one of the basic reasons this book was written. Several examples have been provided in previous chapters. (A discussion on evaluating the satisfactory progression of care will be found in Chapter Eight on "Treatment.")

Here, I would like to focus on non-clinical causes of unsatisfactory care. Among these is the attitude of the physician or other caregivers. If the attitude is haughty, arrogant, uncaring, and/or brusque, the patient is less likely to be pleased, even if the treatment is going as well as possible. If a physician with such negative attitudes errs, he or she can expect little sympathy from patient or family if the question of a malpractice suit arises.

Part of the issue with attitude is the perception by the patient that he or she is not being heard. After all, being heard is the very beginning of any effort at diagnosis or treatment. It's part of the foundation for a positive patient-doctor relationship. And it is certainly the rock-bottom minimum effort that any patient can expect from a physician. The patient needs to continue to be heard throughout the course of treatment. If the doctor comes off as god-like and too "above" the patient to even listen, the patient may be much less forgiving when "god" fails to live up to expectations.

Other than unrealistic expectations, inadequate care, and poor attitude, there are any number of other causes for patient dissatisfaction. No one likes to feel they had to wait excessively long periods to get an appointment, or wait needlessly in the doctor's office. People like to feel that they are treated with respect and courtesy. Most people realize that fees are high (as they are in many fields), but certainly will be offended if they are exorbitant, regardless of who is paying the bills. Additionally, the physician's staff has a large effect on the overall satisfaction or dissatisfaction of the patient. In many ways, the receptionist or switchboard operator lays the first stone in the foundation of the clinical relationship. More blatant causes of dissatisfaction would include sexual inappropriateness on the part of the caregiver, intoxication in the office, obviously unclean equipment, and dishonest billing practices.

Sometimes there is more than enough blame to go around. Obnoxious patients (Type O-Negative "bad patients") are not only more likely to be dissatisfied, they are more likely to be partly responsible for less than optimal results.

No one wins when there is dissatisfaction. Certainly the patient is unhappy and perhaps uncured. The physician finds himself or herself in an uncomfortable position as well. For both parties, the often life-sustaining healing bond between patient and doctor has been weakened, or even completely broken.

. . .

What are some practical steps that can be taken to minimize or correct dissatisfaction? The single most important step is avoiding a set-up for dissatisfaction in the first place. From the instant of the first contact with the physician or office staff, an atmosphere of mutual respect, openness, clear communication, and a shared concern can clear the way for a satisfying relationship and clinical experience.

The patient and the doctor must appreciate each other's limitations. Doctors should understand that patients sometimes are non-compliant; they often will decide to not fully follow instructions. And that they may have trouble understanding what's occurring and need their physician's careful explanations.

Even near the close of the twentieth century, the physician is still the practitioner of an art more than a science. Treatments don't always work. The medical world still has its definite limitations. Physicians should make sure that the patient has a realistic perception of these limitations, without being beaten over the head by them. There are no guarantees, and none should be offered.

If discontentment cannot be prevented, patients and doctors should recognize its development and act promptly to combat it. A simple statement by the patient regarding a concern, followed by a reasonable response from the physician may be all that is required. Unfortunately, patients don't always feel comfortable addressing such a question. And physicians, focusing on the clinical situation, may miss the signs of the patient's displeasure.

In voicing dissatisfaction, the patient may say something like this: "There's a part of this that has been uncomfortable for me, and perhaps has also been uncomfortable for you, doctor." Or, "I feel uncertain about my progress; maybe there is something I don't understand about it." Or, "Could you take a few moments to discuss a concern I have?" Or the physician could start the conversation, saying, "Ms. Smith, I sense you might have a concern about your care. Could we talk about it?"

There are other things that physicians can do if they note dissatisfaction in patients. They need to feel free to speak up and directly address what they see as a possible concern. This should be done in a calm, non-threatening and non-alarmist fashion. It should be at time when the doctor can really sit and listen to the patient. He or she can make an effort to understand the patient's position. Simply debating the issue is rarely helpful or effective.

A next appropriate step might be for the physician to suggest alternative ways in which the current relationship could continue (e.g., with more frequent or longer appointments, or after an outside consultation). Sometimes just talking together about the situation is therapeutic in itself.

If talk does not bring about a resolution, more significant changes may be in order. Options, however, may be somewhat limited due to the patient's circumstances. (Membership in an HMO or financial limitations, for instance.) A patient might even try to educate the physician if he or she has pertinent literature from various support groups.

The patient can ask for a second or even third opinion and ask that the results be sent back to the doctor. Or, if necessary, the patient can consider switching to another physician. It's difficult to know when a patient is acting in his or her own best interest if "doctor hopping" begins. Changing doctors is virtually mandatory if the current situation is headed for disaster. Indeed, the patient has a responsibility to do it. Doctors may not be used to being "fired," but a patient has that right.

But, depending on one's insurance arrangement, unilaterally changing to another physician could prove to be an expensive proposition. Choosing the time for a change of doctors can be somewhat problematic as well. It's difficult to leave in the middle of treatment or during a work-up in progress. Whenever it *is* time, I'd be inclined to find a new physician on my own rather than to ask for a referral from the current doctor. However, the current physician could try to make the transition as smooth as possible. For example, records could be transferred promptly.

A patient might search for other options. Are there alternative types of practitioners available? Perhaps he or she could see a psychologist instead of a psychiatrist, or an optometrist instead of an ophthalmologist.

If you do find yourself dissatisfied or involved in a dispute, you have all the more reason to master as much of the clinical information about your case as possible. Utilize the public library, a local medical library, educational courses, self-help books, and support groups.

If you feel that the provider has violated professional ethics, that there has been demonstrably poor care or that some other impropriety exists, you may wish to contact such authorities as the state licensing board or a professional society of which the physician or other caregiver is a member. Occasionally, legal action appears to be an appropriate response.

. . .

A positive relationship between a patient and physician is not only vital, but it can be one of the most personally rewarding experiences of human life. With such great potential and significance, it's easy to see why the breakdown of this relationship can be so dissatisfying.

Your health is too important to let dissatisfaction stand in the way of improvement—or even survival. Medical care is potentially difficult enough—you do not need the added burden of dissatisfaction and its potentially devastating consequences. Hopefully, your medical involvement has been structured by both you and your physician in such a way as to minimize the risk of such problems. But if discontent does occur, recognize it early, clearly define its nature and deal with it decisively. Hold out as nice of a carrot as you can, but wield as hard of a stick as you must. Get results!

CHAPTER 19

Suing For Malpractice

Pearl:
Justice, compassion, and a desire to improve the system of care can characterize both parties in a malpractice suit.

What this country needs is more medical malpractice suits. It's not that I *like* lawsuits, but they're a valuable option for improving the standards of medical practice. And the volume of poor clinical practice is a blight upon physicians today. There's more malpractice than you can shake a gavel at.

Yes, there is a gain, monetary and otherwise, for the individual patient who wins a suit. But my hope is that all these suits will someday result in substantive changes in how medicine is practiced. Lawsuits keep the issue of quality on the front burner. And if our nation's system of care gets any worse, legal recourse may be almost the last avenue open to force correction.

This chapter will present my position as a physician and as a consumer. Since I'm not an attorney, the following points are simply my thoughts on a significant issue involving my profession. Obviously, this is not a substitute for legal counsel.

Why does malpractice occur in the first place? And why do we have lawsuits resulting from it? These are two quite distinct—but related—issues. Both will be discussed within this chapter.

Medical practice is a very difficult endeavor. Every day, a physician will evaluate thousands of individual bits of data, arriving at hundreds of specific conclusions. Some conclusions will be quite reasonable, but still incorrect. And even the implementation of those conclusions which are correct can be fraught with danger. It's a heavy burden. Juries, sitting on malpractice cases, make their deliberations within this context of reasonable versus unreasonable conclusions, which take place within a very complex environment.

As a practitioner, I don't demand of myself to be always "right," but rather to be reasonable in my actions. If I am knowledgeable, take the time to perform an adequate evaluation, make a thoughtful recommendation, discuss it in detail with the patient who then gives informed consent, I can live with any adverse consequences. Patients, their families, or their attorneys may not be so accepting.

Regardless of who is or isn't satisfied, the existence of a mechanism for bringing malpractice suits is good in theory. If there is an avoidable wrong, some level of compensation is appropriate. And, for every frivolous case brought, there are probably ten valid ones that aren't even recognized as malpractice by the patient or family—and sometimes not even by the physician.

The dollar amounts arrived at in determining the extent of compensation at times appear ludicrous. Judgments can run into the tens of millions of dollars. The process becomes more akin to winning a lottery than achieving justice. I would never argue against just compensation, but determining a price tag for human life and suffering is always arbitrary at best. Must we place it so high, or so arbitrarily, with society bearing the burden of the price tag through higher medical costs?

. . .

The issue of determining blame is an extremely complex one. A negligent act or omission is alleged. This act becomes an isolated "snapshot" of the situation, with the villain framed in the center of the shot.

More often than not, the problem is the result of a long chain of events, rather like a story unfolding in a movie. It is often more rooted in such issues as professional training, efforts to be "cost-effective," facility policies, tradition, or standards of practice (or lack thereof). It really cannot be looked at as a single, isolated, negligent act—except in a court of law.

The real tragedy is how doctors have integrated some of their poor practices along with the unspoken desires, and even mandates, of society. As a nation, we want health care delivered rapidly, cheaply, and to a perfection level of 100 percent. Both physicians and society know that this can't be done, but enter into an unspoken covenant to try. When the god-like doctor breaks the covenant by being caught making an error, then it's time to sue the god.

There is obviously a personal tragedy here for physicians who are successfully sued. To some extent, they are random victims: Many of their colleagues could just as easily been singled out. Their guilt emanates not from a conscious desire to do poorly, but rather from being caught up in practices and approaches which appear to be validated as appropriate by a prestigious profession.

Physicians are sometimes accused of having a conspiracy of silence when it comes to testifying against other physicians in suits. I really don't think that this exists as a conspiracy, but I do think that there is a general reluctance of physicians to testify against each other. They realize that it's often a situation of "there but for the grace of God go I." They recognize the difficulties inherent in practice, and see themselves as being vulnerable to some of the same charges. But a large scale conspiracy? No.

To practice with less legal risk, physicians would have to drastically alter their approach to health care delivery. They would have to train more of their own kind, increasing the number of physicians drastically. These physicians would have to spend increased amounts of time with patients, listening carefully to both their needs and their perceptions of needs. Doctors would have to take the time to develop healing relationships. They would have to recognize both the strengths and limitations of their profession, and make these clear to the patient.

Society would have to expect to pay more to get things done right the first time. But you can make an intelligent argument that doing it right initially would save money in the long run. People would have to start taking responsibility for their own health. They'd have to be willing to become active participants in their health care.

So far, physicians and patients have not been willing to make the necessary changes. That means the guilt is shared between them.

. . .

Regardless of what does or doesn't go wrong with the care, there is a psychology which promotes malpractice suits. Patients and families are often accepting of the fact when something has gone wrong. Additional circumstances may need to occur before a suit will be filed. These include feelings of not being heard, not being allowed to be adequately involved in one's own care and decisions, feelings of not being respected as an individual, and a perception that the treatment was not provided "as advertised." Sometimes patients and doctors simply don't like each other. This is one of the reasons why doctors should strive to work with patients with whom they are well matched and consider referring out those patients with whom they feel they might come into serious conflict.

There are many other possible factors involved in decisions to sue. These include (1) the desire to right a wrong as far as possible, (2) revenge, (3) punishment, (4) wanting appropriate compensation for losses, (5) wanting power or an effort to gain some control, (6) trying to prevent further situations of a similar nature, and (7) giving notice to the profession that this level of care will not be tolerated.

The prominent role of money can not be ignored. After all, "the seat of the psyche is in the wallet." There certainly are greedy patients and greedy lawyers (but then, there are greedy physicians too). And it's generally recognized that we live in a very litigious society: Everyone wants to blame everyone else for everything. For doctors, it's a scary—and expensive—world.

I tell my students that, "A concerned physician gets a cooperative patient—sometimes to the extent of being so cooperative as to not sue when things go wrong." I hope there are more valid reasons for doctors to be concerned than to avoid lawsuits. But I think there are very few physicians who are perceived as concerned who are very often sued.

. . .

What about the malpractice suit itself? A suit, of course, is simply a civil legal action brought by someone who feels wronged (or on behalf of someone who may have been wronged).

Malpractice suits have many nasty characteristics. They tend to get messy, mean, expensive, and time-consuming. And they can become as much of a negative focus for the patient or family as they can for the physician whose whole life can start revolving around issues related to the suit: doubts about competency, concerns over the future, worries over the image presented to patients and colleagues. Likewise, the lives of patients and their families can center around the suit rather than around issues which would relate to care or recovery.

Obviously, malpractice suits are devastating to everyone involved. Do patients have any other alternatives?

Even at the stage of legal involvement, the matter could still be laid to rest with a productive meeting between involved parties. This might include explanations and a discussion of what has been learned by both parties—and no exchange of money. Attorneys may not be happy with such an approach and may even advise against it (they don't make much money this way).

There should be some way of providing compensation that is more beneficial to both the patient and society. Perhaps patients injured during the course of medical treatment should not even have to prove that malpractice occurred. There could be a medical compensation board which would simply make awards based on the occurrence and extent of the injuries, taking into account their impact on the patient's future. Negligence on the part of the physician could be handled by a totally different mechanism, perhaps a licensing review board, or even criminal justice system if appropriate.

Medical compensation could be part of a larger benefits program. A caring society might wish to provide adequate funds to anyone who is injured or disabled within any context, be it auto accidents, work-related injuries, or medical malpractice. This could be done administratively rather than judicially. After all, people will generally be compensated and cared for in one way or another. Why make it more expensive and less productive than it needs to be?

. . .

Unfortunately, such mechanisms for compensating patients are not yet in place. An even better alternative, then, is to avoid malpractice situations in the first place. Naturally, most patients would prefer not be involved in the clinical incidents that result in malpractice, although a few might actually prefer the cash. What can be done to decrease the currently fertile ground for the occurrence of poor care?

Some of these methods have already been mentioned: Train more doctors who are less arrogant and spend more time with patients, while exhibiting a genuine concern. A major role could be played by implementation of the "Four Steps to Better Care." The systematic use of this approach could not only decrease the occurrence of bad practice, but would result in a better relationship between patient and doctor, better care, and more open communication. (Remember that these "Four Steps to Better Care" can be applied by physicians as well as by patients.) Suggestions given in the previous chapter on dissatisfaction can also be used here.

If patients do feel things are amiss, there are a few steps they might take if they are contemplating a lawsuit. Good personal records maintained by the patient can be very helpful in carefully documenting any mistakes and occurrences. With as much material as possible in hand, the patient or family can then more effectively seek legal counsel. Some attorneys specialize in this kind of practice and can be sought out.

. . .

The only real need for malpractice suits is that bad medical care does occur sometimes. This occurrence is obviously not in the interest of the patient, the doctor, nor the institution. In spite of my opening statement in this chapter that more malpractice suits are needed, I hope that in the long run, better practice will mean there will be fewer, if any, needed.

To have less malpractice, physicians will need to change the fundamental ways they try to do "good practice." To have fewer malpractice *cases*, both patients and physicians need to appreciate the limits and uncertainties of clinical care. And physicians should be honest about discussing these in advance. Patients need to participate early in decisions affecting their health.

In the meantime, appropriate suits and awards may give the medical profession the wake-up call it needs.

CHAPTER 20

Assorted Dilemmas

Part Two of this book has dealt with specific practical aspects of health care and its delivery: To be exact, ten topics have been discussed in ten chapters. For obvious reasons, visits to doctors and hospitals have received much of the attention.

In this chapter, I've gathered some additional topics for briefer treatment in a slightly different format. Each section includes a short introduction followed by a numbered list of some insights or hints. They represent what I'd appreciate a physician telling me if I were a lay person dealing with the issue. By no means is the coverage for each topic meant to be comprehensive—only a starting point. But these are additional areas that can't be ignored. If they are of particular concern to you, then continue your research with your physician, with your home or on-line references, at the local book store or public library.

Illness When Traveling

Pearl:
Think of your luggage as your personal traveling health care center, keeping it as well supplied as possible and practical.

A triple whammy is in store for those who develop health problems during a journey. First, there's the same serious need to secure appropriate medical attention or supplies as there would be at home. Secondly, unique practical issues such as language problems, unfamiliarity with local health care resources and problems, and insurance and emergency transportation aspects can become major concerns. Thirdly, the feelings of isolation and anxiety which can accompany almost any illness, can become greater when away (especially if traveling alone)—thereby increasing one's suffering.

Some Major Points

1. If you have known health problems, decide—with your doctor's input—what travel is acceptable and what limitations/precautions are necessary. Do this very early in your planning to help avoid disappointment or changes later on. As always, prevention of problems is primary.
2. The "how, when, where, and with whom" of travel are important health considerations. Some forms of transportation are more physically demanding than others. Even the season of travel can influence your health. The physical environment and its health care resources should be considered. Traveling with a personal companion or relative who could provide some general

assistance may be a good idea. Ships and hotels may either have their own physicians or have access to them.

3. Bring appropriate health care items: extra medications (and written prescriptions), first aid supplies, extra eyeglasses and prescriptions for lenses, a brief written medical history (use Appendix B), basic over-the-counter drugs, thermometer, and insurance information. Travel with as many of these as practical. What's easily obtainable at home may be very difficult to come by overseas or even in the U.S. at 3 a.m. Don't pack prescription medications in checked baggage. Do divide up your prescription between bags you are personally carrying. For example, put half in your purse or briefcase and half in your carry-on bag.

4. Do as much advance planning as possible. A number of organizations and reference sources provide information or insurance coverage related to such travel issues as: emergency air evacuation, availability of physicians and facilities, immunizations, medical records, and health risks. Travel agents may be able to assist with a number of these. The Centers for Disease Control in Atlanta can be a useful source for some of this information. Except for the cost of the phone call, you can access their voice information system free of charge at (404)332-4555. I found this system quite complex as I worked my way through the menus; be prepared with a pen and paper when you dial. Also check out what your library has available on travel and health.

5. Always carry a general medical guide with you. For me, it's the *Merck Manual.* You might want to get something lighter in weight and style. But I consider it essential to have a printed resource available.

6. Call your home physician for basic guidance when problems arise during travel. Even overseas calls aren't that expensive compared to the value of your health. Don't expect a diagnosis over the phone, but the general advice provided could be extremely useful.

7. Avoid situations which carry a high risk of illnesses, injuries, or assaults —for example, don't plan on running with the bulls in Spain. Also inquire carefully about the water quality. Be a smart traveler, remaining extra-vigilant when away from familiar home turf. The further away you are, the greater the vigilance. Again, prevention is the key word.

8. For psychological as well as physical well-being, try to keep a reasonable sameness in routine without denying yourself some of the spontaneity and novelty of travel. Eat meals on a regular schedule, sleep at the usual times, stick to exercise routines, don't overdo strenuous activities, and do schedule in some of your usual relaxations such as reading, walking, or watching TV.

9. Have a "plan B" if all else fails. You're away, you're ill, and there are no adequate local health care resources to tap into. What are your options? Consider them before a health problem develops. This is especially true if you have a chronic illness where you might anticipate both the occurrence and nature of the difficulty. For example, in truly isolated areas, do you have some means of communication with the outside world? Do you know enough first-aid to adequately attend to your own injuries? Do you have adequate financial resources? While travel on the proverbial shoestring can sound romantic and adventuresome, such pleasures can soon fade when faced with the necessity for hard cash during a medical emergency.

10. For the sake of your mental health, keep your expectations reasonable. Travel isn't always a wonderful voyage of discovery. It can be tiring, frustrating, anxiety-provoking, and disappointing.

    Carefully weigh all the risks and benefits of travel. Don't automatically deny yourself the joys of travel simply because of a health problem. But don't put your health and life in jeopardy just because of a desire to travel. Think of travel as a stretching of your metaphorical umbilical cord. The further you are from home, the thinner is the cord attaching you to your usual resources and to the familiar.

If travel is a reasonable choice for you, then plan carefully, act cautiously—and enjoy!

. . .

Considering Nursing Home Care

Pearl:
The term "nursing home" is a euphemism.

Personally, I'd rather live in a place called an "old-folks home" than in a "nursing home." Somehow it seems more honest and hopeful. At least I'd be with other "old-folks" rather than being "nursed."

There are three major issues to consider in regard to nursing homes: (1) the role of modern societal changes, (2) the characteristics of quality facilities, and (3) guilt.

Part of the reason for increasingly placing elderly or disabled family members outside the home has been the marked changes within the family and the community. "Mom" has not only become old and sick, she has unfortunately done so in our modern society. From a practical standpoint, care at home with the family may no longer be seen as a viable option. It strikes me as interesting that day care for children may be seen as the other side of the coin of nursing home care for a primarily elderly population.

With this increased need for care, there are more and more facilities actively marketing themselves. But you can largely ignore any slick promotional material. Such literature is frequently more closely related to marketing goals than to reality. Instead, you should pay attention to the facility itself.

In evaluating a nursing home, look first for the obvious things: cleanliness, appearance, food, staff availability, accommodations, and costs. Then look at less apparent aspects: activity programs, medical services, staff experience and training, and social service resources. Equally important are the attitude of the staff toward each other and toward the residents, as well as your own "gut feeling" of what you observe.

Once the decision to place a loved one has been made and an appropriate facility has been chosen, families often have to contend with guilt over a number of issues: Was a nursing home really necessary? Could I have done more? Am I contributing enough?

Nursing home placement can be a painful, gut-wrenching, often divisive, experience for families. The following tips, implemented before and after placement, may help alleviate some of those feelings.

Some Major Points

1. Ideally, family members and the prospective nursing home resident should discuss preferences and arrangements far in advance of any actual need. Often, the move can be anticipated months or even years ahead of time.

2. Frequently, there's disagreement among family members. Each should be allowed to make his or her own particular case. This could include a statement of the personal and monetary contributions each individual would be willing to make. Every effort should be made to reach a consensus. "Dumping" on any particular family member or members is obviously less preferable than is a shared responsibility.

3. Consideration of a wide range of alternatives may be helpful. These would include such options as live-in help; placing the individual in a willing family member's home, with other family members agreeing to help out; home health care; or adult day care.

4. Get recommendations and general information from others who have placed family members in facilities.

5. Visit a reasonable number of facilities to get a sense of their strengths and weaknesses. People sometimes spend months house-hunting, during which time they see numerous residences. A search for a nursing home also deserves a similarly serious effort.

6. Weigh heavily geographical proximity to family members as a major factor in selection. As with house-hunting, location is extremely important.

7. Talk to patients and staff, not just administrators. Remember, it's the administration's job to sell the facility.

8. Once the person is admitted, be as actively involved in the care as possible and/or necessary, taking into account the wishes and independence of that person. Inquire, with permission of the resident if indicated,

about medications and any restraining devices which may be used (for instance, special chairs or belts—ask the staff to show you what these look like and under what circumstances they would be used).

9. Consider volunteering at the facility. It provides an opportunity for a personal charitable activity, and it allows for additional contact with the family member while simultaneously keeping an eye on the operation of the facility.

10. Keep the individual as actively involved in the family as possible.

11. Don't look to placement to necessarily resolve or improve relationships between the resident and the family or between the family members themselves. Such improvement may take additional effort and discussion.

A decision for nursing home placement is rarely easy. But the situation can often be made more palatable for the individual and less painful for the family. Careful planning, adequate discussion, common sense, and a solid, loving relationship built over the years, can carry the day.

. . .

Rural Health Care

Pearl:

In this age of instant communication and modern transportation, "rural" is more of a state-of-mind than a geographic location.

Discussions of rural health care often focus on weaknesses rather than on its strengths. It's true that rural areas often have problems in terms of availability of facilities as well as the presence of adequately trained professional staff. But hospitals in isolated areas often make up in personal attention what they lack in physical facilities and variety of staff. This can increase the probability of appropriate care. There must be some reason that there are so many healthy farmers, ranchers, and their families out there in rural America.

Some additional pluses of rural care should be noted. In these areas, there is an awareness of a significant health care delivery problem which, in itself, helps deal with that problem. Rural areas aren't likely to take care for granted. They often have well-organized emergency response services which allow for quicker action to compensate for the increased distances. Rural areas also may have both formal and informal care networks with facilities in nearby population centers.

More physicians will move into rural areas if two things occur. First, an increased supply of doctors in metropolitan areas would provide a market force helping to shift them into more needy parts of the country. Second, seeing the recreational and family advantages that many rural areas offer could be an extremely positive force in encouraging medical migration.

Medically needy rural communities could do much to organize their part of the delivery system: Become more cooperative in developing regional rather than local facilities, provide quality emergency services, and arrange pooled transportation for routine medical visits to more distant centers. Medical schools could do their part by emphasizing rural health care and providing students with clinical experience in these areas.

Some Major Points

1. Rural communities often have the ability to be more manageable and to pull together more effectively in making health care changes than do larger population centers. They may have more flexibility and a more focused desire to work effectively.

2. Rural health care is becoming a more fashionable issue and we'll all be hearing a lot more about it, especially in the political arena.

3. Small regional multi-specialty clinics might serve needs better than having solo practitioners scattered randomly around the rural areas. Speaking personally as one who has been there, I would much rather practice as a specialist in a small group serving a region than as a family physician, solo or otherwise, serving a single small town. And I think I would thereby serve the needs of the community better. Such an approach could also have linked to it supportive arrangements with other nearby regional groups and more distant metropolitan centers.

4. Family doctors could serve the rural community better by being more like "first-line health defenders," referral sources, and family medical advisors. This would remove them from their current, more interventionist role of being a supermarket for all types of care. I fear that many are poorly equipped to deliver some services when they try to offer so much. "Jack of all trades" is a concept that doesn't work as well in health care.

5. A focus on prevention is especially important in rural environments because of the dangers of farm implement accidents and chemical hazards, as well as because of the lesser availability of services once problems arise.

6. Health care personnel such as midwives, nurse practitioners, dentists, optometrists, and podiatrists could be utilized to a fuller advantage. There should be an upfront understanding as to abilities and limitations. An especially controversial topic is to what extent some of these professionals should be allowed to do work

more traditionally associated with physicians. Much of the hesitation by the medical establishment to support increased participation is quite legitimate; at other times it's merely a "turf" issue. At a minimum, until physicians are willing to replicate themselves in large enough numbers (and then move to serve these areas), I feel strongly that those who are willing and otherwise able be allowed to fill the need.

7. Make rural (and inner-city) service mandatory for those medical students benefiting from government funding. These special environments could be settings for their training as well as required sites of later temporary practice in order to provide a payback for their education.

America's rural population deserves as high a level of quality care as anyone. This isn't likely to be achieved within the current structure and attitudes of the medical world. But, significant positive changes, as presented above, could come without overwhelming expenses.

. . .

Using Clinics and Mega-Clinics

Pearl:

Regardless of the kind of medical facility you use, good care at its most basic level comes down to one good doctor and one good patient working together.

In science fiction literature, characters can sometimes change shape to assume a variety of forms. That's a good analogy to keep in mind when trying to understand the concept of "clinics."

A clinic can be a one-doctor office or a complex mega-structure with many hundreds of physicians. It can be an extensive mecca of cutting-edge technology or a store-front operation barely adequate for basic services. In fact, the term "clinic" is often associated with free or low-cost public facilities which are typically less than state-of-the-art.

Some clinics are multi-specialty organizations which are known for diagnostic expertise and sophisticated procedures (like the Mayo Clinic). Others are more associated with single specialties such as psychiatry (the Menninger Clinic), still others are known primarily for work with a single illness (the Joslin Diabetes Center), or even a single symptom such as headache or depression.

To confuse things even more, some clinics are like the mythical Brigadoon in the musical of the same name: They appear and disappear at intervals. They use borrowed offices where they hang up their shingle only while in session. When the session is over, the clinic is gone.

Even at the more famous clinics in the U.S., not everyone leaves cured or even satisfied. Big isn't necessarily better, but size can often bring together the specialists, equipment, and other resources which can lead to success where others have failed.

Other issues to consider regarding clinics:

Some Major Points

1. Be sure you understand the nature of a clinic before you visit. Learn as much about it as possible.

2. Within a reasonably short distance of almost anyone there will be a multi-specialty clinic. For difficult cases and special needs, these can be lifesavers. Ask your physician or consult available directories. The American Medical Group Association (703)838-0033 can provide locations.

3. At some clinics you might feel somewhat adrift because the facility staff may look upon its patients as having a relationship with the clinic rather than with a particular doctor. Patients who affiliate themselves with a clinic should define the relationship between themselves, the physicians they are seeing, and the clinic.
4. Don't be awed by grandeur. Big and well-known won't always translate into success for the patient. The patient may have to be just as vigilant at a mega-clinic as elsewhere. There will still be the necessity of keeping in mind the "Four Steps to Better Care."
5. Don't accept indifferent and inadequate care at the reduced-cost or free clinics. Regardless of what a patient is paying (or not paying), the same level of courtesy and quality is appropriate. That quality may be limited by the clinic's resources, but this should be explained to the patient.

. . .

Terminal Illness

Pearl:

No matter how serious the problem, there are always some options.

It would be better if terminal (fatal) illnesses could be reserved for the "pros" amongst patients—those with more experience in dealing with the medical world. Unfortunately, things don't always work that way. On any given day, any of us could find that we are "terminal." It's a very difficult situation, but the following points may help.

Some Major Points

1. A terminal illness used to be a profoundly personal event. In this modern world, much of its significance has been converted to a medical event—or even a series of medical events. The focus is often away from the individual and on the technology. How much is being done is measured by the number of machines and medications rather than by the depth of the caring.

2. Psychological aspects of terminal illnesses are often worse than their physical aspects. The fear, anxiety, isolation, and depression can be far, far worse than the pain or other physical symptoms.

3. Preparation *is* possible. People who live meaningful lives are better prepared to face terminal illness and prepare for a "good" death. The object of life is not, after all, to live as long as possible. It's to live as well as possible, within the context of how we define the meaning of our own lives. If we prepare for death to have as much meaning as our lives, we can cope more effectively during a crisis.

4. Even with a terminal illness, there are always options. These may include palliative (non-curative, but beneficial) care, further efforts at cure (even if it is against the odds), or non-traditional treatments. They also include non-clinical options such as how a patient can make use of his or her remaining time: including making peace with oneself or one's family and friends, drawing up a will, attending to unfinished business, and deciding

where and with whom one might wish to die. Some patients and families feel more comfortable if the final setting is in a hospital, others prefer a hospice, still others prefer to be home.

5. Of course, the patient will want to make sure that he or she truly is terminal. It does happen that patients are given an incorrect diagnosis. A second (or even third) opinion may cast new light on this situation.

6. Hope is a state of mind of which people should never be deprived. The hope may be that they can successfully survive the illness, accomplish their goals before death, or even have a miraculous recovery. I don't think it's ever the right of anyone to deprive the patient of some hope. This is not to imply that physicians or family should mislead a patient, but that they shouldn't try to remove all hope since none of us are given absolutely certain knowledge of the future. For some, religious faith provides strength and hope. These patients who are hospitalized may wish to take advantage of chaplaincy services.

7. As with religion, philosophy may become a very important issue for people during a terminal illness. They may wish to use this intellectual discipline to make sense of their lives and their impending death.

8. We don't usually think of psychiatric illnesses as terminal. But there are a significant number of the mentally ill who commit suicide, and there are some who suffer fatal reactions to medications. Other patients' lives are so chronically and seemingly permanently disrupted by debilitating mental illness that, for all intents and purposes, they might as well be considered within this terminal group.

We occasionally hear talk of "beating" a terminal illness. Perhaps some people do it by willpower or by some other unknown strength. But most of us will be doing well to simply deal with a terminal illness with acceptance and dignity. I think it is usually more a matter of the person's spirit not being beaten by an illness rather than of that person beating it.

Is there a "silver lining" in having a terminal illness? I suppose it depends on one's perspective. Would you rather have the forewarning of a terminal illness so as to finish up your earthly business and prepare for death? Or would you rather die unsuspectingly in your sleep, with no such warning?

. . .

Death, the Inevitable Ending

Pearl:
We may not be able to control when we go, but we can often influence under what circumstances.

This section focuses more on events related to the very end of a terminal illness: death.

As surely as our bodies are programmed to start breathing after birth, they are already programmed to start dying. Processes are set in motion at conception which will inevitably result in our "natural" death—if injuries or other potentially avoidable problems don't intervene first.

Death is rightly or wrongly often seen by doctors and layperson alike as our major enemy. A number of factors contribute to this perception:

1. Death will always be the great unknown ("near-death" experiences not withstanding).

2. People have an exceedingly strong instinct for survival.
3. Many people believe that after death there is nothing—and, therefore, that they will be nothing.
4. Warding off death is the most important power perceived to be held by physicians.

Death is almost as complicated as life. It's logistically quite messy. That's why any possible preparation is important. These days, it's accepted that hospitals already start planning patients' discharges on the day they're admitted. Perhaps we should all take a cue from this and start our own "ultimate discharge planning" as early in our lives as we can.

Some Major Points

1. The way we live can greatly influence the way we die. To be comfortable with life can allow one to accept death more comfortably. Death is the natural and normal progression of life. We can learn to deal with death through our life's experiences. Our involvement with the deaths of family members and friends (and even pets) is both painful and valuable. Thinking of death shouldn't be confined to times of our illnesses, terminal or not. People in their 20s and 30s plan for retirement. Perhaps they should do some thinking about their deaths as well.
2. There are many psycho-philosophical issues for those facing death. These include the value people see in friends and relatives—and the strength which can subsequently be drawn from them in one's last moments. People must value their own deaths. In much the same

way, society must value the death of each of its members. Even the most uncomfortable of deaths can be accomplished with dignity if that dignity is inherent within the person.

3. There are some times that we can influence <u>when</u> death will occur. There may be an order from the doctor of "D.N.R." (do not resuscitate) when prolongation of life would be misguided. A durable power of attorney for health care can direct those you trust so that they can make critical decisions when you are unable to. A Living Will is another advance directive which helps to make your wishes known.

4. Suicide or assisted-suicide is felt by some to be an option. This is obviously a very controversial issue. I can only say that I see all human lives—even painful and desperate ones—as having value. In any case, our society may ultimately wish to have "executioners," but I don't feel that physicians should play this role in assisted suicide. Nor do I see the physician's role as one of artificially maintaining a life whose natural end has come. Sometimes overlooked is the fact that death can even be surprisingly welcome to the patient (and, perhaps, even appropriately by the family).

5. If you're asked to consent to an autopsy for a family member, inquire as to the specific information likely to result from it. If you have questions which are unanswered regarding someone's death, get input from a physician regarding whether or not an autopsy would help resolve them.

6. Most of us are taught that there is a value to everyday life. Death, also, is not without its value—even when

> the end seems tragic or apparently meaningless. The meaning may simply be to validate us as a civilized people as we provide proper care to the dying.

Our challenge is to meet death rather than succumb to it. We can do this with dignity and wisdom. Our last days—even if spent in increased suffering—can be our best.

. . .

Part One of this book has tried to pass on some basic understanding of what influences the health care system and how that system actually operates. Part Two has focused largely on practical applications of that material to your care.

Now it's time to take stock and to plan for the future. What is the outlook—the prognosis, in medical lingo—for our own health care and for that of our nation's health care delivery system?

Onward to Part Three. You'll see that the prognosis depends very much on *you*.

PART 3

Prognosis

CHAPTER 21

What's Worth Saving in Modern Medicine?

Pearl:
Health care dollars are better spent on human resources than on "bricks and mortar."

America remains a throw-away society. If it's old or doesn't work perfectly, we're just as likely to toss it out as to fix it. But we can't afford this approach in health care.

You know by now that I am not enamored with health care as it is currently delivered in the U.S. Yet even I would be reluctant to just say, "Toss it!" A too-rapid revamp would be equally unacceptable. First of all, we have so much that is actually good. Second, what would we be getting in exchange? In addition, with just about everything in the Biz-Med Complex connected to everything else, changes can cause tremendous and unforeseeable ripple effects. We're going to have to recycle.

You could probably compile a reasonable list of medicine's more positive aspects right now. But, unless you actually perform such an unlikely exercise, the obvious is easily overlooked.

The airline industry can provide a useful comparative study. It's somewhat better defined than the more sprawling and amorphous health care industry. And, considering the complexity of its task, commercial aviation can claim a better safety record than can health care.

Planes efficiently move masses of people daily in relative safety and comfort for generally reasonable charges. Still, flying has its annoyances and—rarely—its spectacular tragedies. But the industry also has a large fleet, convenient schedules, skilled pilots, an extensive training program, an efficient air traffic control system, rigorous maintenance, and generally pleasant personnel.

Recognizing these strengths helps us to be more comfortable when we board an aircraft. We understand the industry better, and as a result, perhaps we gripe about it less. We can also see that there's a solid base from which future change and further improvement can be made.

Health care is much like this. We feel reasonably safe interacting within the system. And when we recognize its assets, we get a broader perspective and can see a better foundation for more improvement.

Actually, modern health care has a lot going for it. The system is not really so bad, it's just that it is so much less good than it might be. On a scale of 1 to 10, I would give it a "7" (perhaps somewhat generously). There are a few parts of our society which we would especially like to see come in as "10s." Health care is one of these. I'd put the airline industry at a "9."

So let's list health care's assets, the parts worth saving. They range in nature from the psychological to the structural.

Modern facilities and technology: In the U.S., almost everyone is already reasonably close to some inpatient or outpatient facility. Our country is in the forefront of the "bricks and mortar" aspect of health care. (The quality delivered once the patient arrives may be another issue.) We are similarly blessed with an ever-expanding technological alphabet soup of helpful technology: EEG, MRI, PSA, and CAT scan to name a few.

As health care has become more entrepreneurial, we're even experiencing some medical sprawl as both small and large provider organizations establish outposts, bringing their technology with them. These could be utilized more if clinics operated on an expanded schedule of 7 a.m. to 10 p.m. In addition, expensive hospital diagnostic equipment could run almost 24 hours a day. But for now, at least the facilities and the equipment are in place.

The distinction between outpatient and inpatient facilities is diminishing. Hospitals are providing more and more outpatient services. And outpatient facilities are doing more surgery.

Patients have more choices today. These can range from the walk-in doc-in-a-box, or the traditional solo office of the family doctor, to small groups practices and mega-clinics. Individuals, communities, and businesses have committed huge investments in these various facilities.

Perhaps the biggest failing among facilities is a lack of integration with other parts of the system. The inadequacies of networking hinders patients within one part of the system from routinely reaping the benefits existing in other parts—even just across the town or across the street.

Treatments: If "miracle" is too strong a word for some of the treatments available today, it doesn't miss by much. We can open up the clogged arteries of a heart or even replace the heart itself. Bone marrow transplants, antipsychotic medications, help for infertile couples, blood transfusion, a plethora of antibiotics to fight infection, radiation therapy for tumors—the list seems endless. We are blessed!

But there are problems: Not everyone has access to all the "miracles;" physicians sometimes prescribe them inappropriately; patients are too often prevented from fully participating in their care in appropriate ways; and—as in the case of parents neglecting to have their children immunized—people too frequently fail to take advantage of what is available.

Transportation: Sometimes the speed with which a patient is transported to a facility and the efficiency of the facility when the patient arrives are more important factors than the patient's actual distance from the facility. An accident victim who cannot be reached by emergency crews because of a clogged urban expressway may be no better off than an injured farmer 50 miles from the closest hospital over open country roads.

We're blessed with many well-trained and well-equipped ambulance crews, not to mention helicopters and fixed-wing aircraft that are used for medical transportation. Many emergency services and vehicles are the result of monetary donations and numerous hours of volunteer time. In instances of extensive disasters, we have assistance from support organizations such as the Red Cross and Salvation Army. What we are lacking is an extensive formal network for transporting people—especially the elderly—for *routine* care.

Professionals: Millions of health care professionals stand ready to care for us. Patients arriving for emergency care are often efficiently triaged; that is, sorted out in order of their need to receive attention. Usually they'll find a knowledgeable staff on hand to provide care. Rarely are people turned away from the critical care they need.

Patients seeking out less urgent care will find a diversity of trained professionals. An army of physicians, physicians' assistants, nurse practitioners, midwives, technicians, psychologists, dentists, social workers, pharmacists, optometrists, and other healthcare providers stand ready to provide services.

Training: Health care professionals typically have long and arduous educational requirements. Not only are programs already in place in an extensive network of training institutions, but these programs could be expanded to accommodate a larger number of women, minorities, and other people who would apply if they were encouraged to do so. Much of medical education is provided at no cost by volunteer teachers. While our educational system is extremely inefficient, the potential is there for improvement with limited expenditure.

Research: Health care professionals practice upon a foundation of scientific research developed over the centuries. Much of it is excellent. Recent concern over the conduct of studies on breast cancer is an example of potential problems within the scientific community. Despite its weak links, research has brought us miracle drugs and miraculous surgeries. Such efforts receive tremendous assistance from universities, government, private industry, and philanthropic foundations.

Support: There's a nearly invisible "army" with a massive supply corps to back up the front-line caregivers and myriad activities of health care. Administrators, firms providing medical supplies, pharmaceutical companies, and many others make modern health care deliverable. They often thrive by tapping into our country's entrepreneurial spirit.

Variety/choice: While patients often have limitations regarding who they see for care, where they are seen, and when they are seen, there is also opportunity for choice. Patients can choose from numerous hospitals and clinics, group practices and solo practices, specialists and generalists, health care plans, growing numbers of "mid-level" practitioners, and even "alternative" medical care.

The patient-doctor relationship: Not everyone has a strong, positive, therapeutic relationship with their physician. But where this does exist, it can be marvelous to behold. To what extent will future changes in health care result in patients and doctors becoming more adversarial than we are already starting to see? To what extent will changes weaken the healing bonds that have developed?

Positive attitudes: This is one of the most important of all the categories mentioned. People with positive attitudes are our real strength. Without them, the rest may not matter. Many providers want to be generous, caring, and compassionate. This isn't always easy in our modern society. It's hard for people to rise above the background noise of excessive profits and self-centeredness. But within the Biz-Med Complex there are many dedicated practitioners, business people, and workers who really do try. We need them all.

. . .

Some of the above resources are not available to every person all the time. They may require major improvement, expansion, or even redefining. Nonetheless, they are there. They provide a viable foundation upon which to build a more effective and responsive system.

At this point, we cannot afford to reinvent the health care wheel. While saving the good that we have, we can make changes and additions which are both meaningful and substantive.

We have a responsibility to protect our useful resources. While we may reinvent our philosophical approaches to health care, we can only hope to redevelop our current assets. With this almost embarrassment of riches, the real question becomes, "Why are we using them so poorly?"

CHAPTER 22

Our Society and the Future of Health Care

Pearl:
Our system of health care is a major part of the yardstick which measures us as a society.

Health care has become so intertwined with our society that it has become nearly impossible to separate the two. Executions are becoming clinical as well as punitive procedures. Violence may be genetic and consequently defined as a medical problem. Drug abuse is an illness. Veterans may function inadequately in our society because they have Posttraumatic Stress Disorder. Abortion is an issue between patient and doctor. Ownership of handguns has become a public health issue. Homosexuality is an alternative lifestyle because many psychiatrists say so. Dr. Kevorkian can help you kill yourself. Soon, the question of ending the life of the suffering elderly, even without their assistance, may move into the public arena for active consideration.

As our society becomes more complex and distressed, will professionals simply diagnose those unable to adjust as having a "modern world syndrome?" Will we thereby further medicalize our failings and further reduce personal responsibility?

The question here is, "What is appropriate clinical involvement?" Are health care professionals assuming power by claiming expertise beyond acceptable limits? Is society looking for "experts" to justify its actions? On the surface, at least, it appears that the medical world has become our mouthpiece when society is unable to speak for itself.

An argument could certainly be made that, regardless of the reason, the effect is the same: Society has shifted much of its decision-making to the clinicians. At a minimum, people need to recognize the implications of this. They need to ask if clinicians have become the saviors or the scapegoats of our society. Health care professionals should ask themselves if they have identified society's victims or have they created them. Everyone needs to ask what will happen if government begins to take over more and more of health care and its decision-making.

The more technologically advanced our society becomes, the more decision-making power caregivers will have. The basic formula is simple: Because we have the technology, we use it. Because we use it, we proclaim it "good."

But not every situation is a medical situation. My message here is primarily one of *awareness*. If "medicalization" is what we want, let's at least acknowledge what's happening and study our agreement. Until then, professional caregivers should be devoted servants of society, not its masters by default or coup.

. . .

The world has a number of two-way streets. For example, the more economic disruption we have, the more crime we have, and vise versa. The road between society and the health care community is one of the broader boulevards. Not only does health care influence society, society very much influences health care. For all of its strengths, our health care system does have its serious problems. Many of these are tied to the problems of our society as a whole.

Physicians and other health care workers come from the same population pool as dedicated teachers, honest laborers, and valiant soldiers. But also in that pool are crooked bankers, inside traders, spouse-abusers, and excessive drinkers. Those entering the medical world bring with them the strengths *and* the baggage of that larger society.

While there will always be a resonance between society and health care, should either take precedence over the other in ethical and moral leadership? It appears that the medical world has been given permission to do exactly that. Most people seem comfortable with this.

I believe health care professionals have largely failed in this expectation of excellence. This book is replete with examples. But what can be done? The needed reform can come either from inside or outside of the profession. Professionals, after using their talents and resources to clean up their own act, could turn these to providing a more productive and ideal relationship between them and society.

To what extent can society itself substantively change? Philosophers and sociologists could argue this endlessly. From a purely pragmatic view point, I would argue that society can not only change, but that it *must*—and fast. And not just in the area of health care.

Or, of course, the government could regulate from the outside. But such regulation is similar to attacking crime by focusing on building more prisons instead of dealing with the causes of criminal behavior. Whether the issue is crime or health care, only a temporary and superficial benefit—at best—occurs as a result of more governmental manipulation.

. . .

If we are going to continue to have any type of an honorable and productive alliance between society and the health care system, there will be some prerequisites:

1. Effective, active, positive leadership from both sides.
2. A more professional (and all that word implies) delivery system provided by the medical world.
3. The fullest possible expression of the "Four Steps to Better Care" as it can be applied by both patients and caregivers.
4. Strong personal ethical commitments by professionals and laypeople alike.

One aspect of the task is to ask this as a society: "What do we want from modern medicine?" Perhaps part of the answer is that we want it to deliver a product which is at least as efficient as those delivered by airlines or by express package delivery services, for instance. But we must be cautious to make the distinction between having medicine operate as efficiently as some businesses, and having it actually be more of a business. As I stressed in the first chapter of this book, we need to move from the current Biz-Med Complex model, which has a largely financial base, to one which is focused more on professionalism.

If such a shift were accomplished, I would suspect that a stabilization or even decrease in cost might occur. Even if it didn't, I doubt that most Americans would object since real value would likely result from increased leadership and improved care.

. . .

In the first chapter in this book I introduced the "Four Steps to Better Care." These are not only an individual's guide to personal health care. They can also have an application to our individual roles in society and to the larger health care system which is part of that society. Allow me to cast them in a broader context:

1. Understanding: includes the need for everyone, including professionals, to know themselves, their communities, and their health care delivery system—and the resulting interactions.

2. Involvement: means professionals, non-professionals, and governmental and private organizations working to actively shape both society and health care in productive ways.

3. Responsibility: befalls all who are capable of being involved; that is, almost every adult. This is not discretionary, but obligatory.

4. Authority: to make appropriate decisions and accomplish production change is a right which accompanies the responsibility. Such authority would be guided by both law and ethics.

A book such as this can help empower individuals to apply these "Four Steps to Better Care" to their personal health care. However, it can take very strong leadership inside and outside of the health care field to empower our society to implement these steps as a nation.

Regardless of how productive or disastrous their association may be, society and health care cannot help being actively linked together. They share a future influenced by each other's progress and failings.

CHAPTER 23

A Dozen Practical Steps You Can Take Today

Pearl:

Aspirin and a Merck Manual are two of the best values in health care today—but both still have to be used appropriately.

Change rarely comes easily, and this book asks that you markedly change your approach to health care. Having a list of specific tasks—especially ones that can be done right away—can help you get started.

The following is a practical, straightforward list of 12 steps you can take now. Most of the items require no significant expenditure of either time or money. Those that do can be well worth the investment. Why not use these twelve points as a checklist, marking off each one as it's accomplished?

1. *Buy two family medical reference books.* There are a number of useful family medical guides on the market. Browse through the selections at your local bookstore and see what suits you. I won't make any specific recommendations other than to suggest that you buy not one,

but two. (The Mayo Clinic even has a family guide on CD-ROM!)

The advantage of two references are many. Health care is a serious enough endeavor to have a cross-reference available. With regard to specific information, one book may have what you are seeking while the other one won't. One may be more readable than the other in certain sections. They may provide different approaches to care. And if you read the same information in two different texts, you can have a little bit more faith in its validity.

Also, if you have a chronic illness such as asthma, diabetes, or high blood pressure; get yet another book—a guide for non-professionals entirely devoted to your problem.

2. *Buy a Merck Manual.* A *Merck Manual* is really the "doctor's bible." This marvelous little book is updated with a new edition about every five years. The 1992 edition runs almost 3,000 pages and costs about $25. I value mine so much that I pack it in my luggage every time I take a trip.

   Yes, it is written for the professional, but it is well-written. I think that the average person who wanted to know about the most current approach of the medical world to a specific problem would do well to refer to this text. While every word may not be understood, the general thrust of diagnosis and treatment of particular problems will likely come through.

   You can use the *Merck Manual* in conjunction with (probably after) reading your patient-guides. And—of course—you can ask your doctor to clarify things you don't understand. (A guidebook on medications would make a nice fourth addition to your medical library.)

3. *Make an appointment for a routine exam and to "diagnose" your doctor.* If you've just moved or are otherwise in the process of changing doctors, this is a good time to make an appointment just to get to know your new physician. Although it may also be an opportunity for a general check-up, this wouldn't be absolutely necessary. Make at least a 15-minute appointment to go in, get acquainted, let the doctor get acquainted with you, and ask him or her some of the questions that have been discussed in Chapter 10 about the doctors appointment. See how you like the doctor's style. Make an evaluation as to whether or not you'd be comfortable with this practitioner.

   Here are some very open-ended questions to get you started:

   - "What's your general 'style' of practice—would you say it's aggressive or conservative?"
   - "How, specifically, do you work with patients with regard to emergencies? With regard to calls to be seen that day? With regard to calls requesting advice over the phone?"

   You can also come up with your own questions which reflect your particular concerns. (I think physicians should offer visits for the sole purpose of "getting-acquainted" without charge or perhaps at a very minimal fee.)

4. *Ask three friends or neighbors to name the best doctor and the best hospital they know.* Ask them, "why?" Even if you think you do know who to see, ask anyway.

If you personally know some nurses poll them on who they feel is the best doctor. I don't know of any better source of accurate information on the quality of physicians, their strengths and weaknesses.

While you're talking to nurses or friends, ask about hospitals as well. Be aware that nurses currently working at a particular facility may be less than objective.

5. *Request your medical records.* Patients can benefit from having a copy of their own medical records at home. They are not only for enhancing your own understanding, but also in providing information as the need arises. (Also, copy and complete the medical history form found in Appendix B.)

   Send a letter to your doctor's office requesting your records be photocopied and sent to you. There may be a charge for this, so ask first. A doctor might actually feel somewhat threatened because of such a request. He or she may think you may have some suspicion about them, or may even be contemplating a lawsuit. So explain your innocent intentions if you feel it will ease the situation. The kind of response you get to your request—or lack thereof—may be quite informative in itself!

6. *Lower your expectations for health care.* Make a decision to recognize the limitations of modern health care. Every discomfort, illness, and uncertainty will not necessarily find a quick resolution in the medical community. This isn't said to discourage you from seeking appropriate attention when indicated. However, early or intermittent symptoms cannot always be diagnosed; hidden disease will not always be detected. Diagnoses aren't always accurate, especially when they

involve psychiatric labels. Working your way through the system may be tedious and aggravating. Health care is not a cure-all. You can lower your frustration level by being realistic about your expectations.

7. *Start following simple basic health and safety rules*. These are almost too well-known to mention in any detail here. Healthwise, eat a nutritious diet; exercise regularly; avoid smoking; avoid excessive intake of alcohol and inappropriate use of other drugs; deal reasonably with emotional stress and conflicts; see your physician for routine care as well as for emerging problems as indicated; and if you are in agreement with your doctor's proposed treatment program for you, follow it carefully. If you're not in agreement, maybe it's time for a second opinion.

   Following simple basic safety rules is similarly important. There are many ways of avoiding "accidents." In a way, some occurrences can hardly be classified as accidents because they are so easily preventable. You needn't be a rocket scientist to know to leave a golf course during a thunderstorm or to lock up medicine. Utilize a generally cautious attitude—but not timidity—in your life. Be your own best "risk manager."

8. *Read any material you have on your health care benefits*. Do you know your health care benefits? Do you know what coverage is available for mental health care? What about obstetrical coverage? How are medications and outpatients visits covered? Does your coverage pay for a second opinion? I realize that the printed material you may have regarding your coverage may not be user-friendly. You may need an interpreter; your agent or employer may be able to help.

You should know what your insurance covers for at least three reasons: (1) so that you can consider changing the coverage if you feel it's inadequate, (2) to take appropriate advantage of the coverage you do have, and (3) to be prepared to handle expenses not covered. When an illness has already occurred, it is not the time to be surprised by limitations of your insurance benefits.

9. *Resolve to focus on living well rather than living long.* (There is no prize for mere longevity, especially for a long and dissatisfying life.) In spite of how emphatic this book may be at times, I am by no means suggesting a rigid regimentation of a person's life for the sole purpose of improving health care. Health care is only a part of life—it's not life itself.

   It's perfectly acceptable for people to want to enjoy food, to be reasonably adventuresome, and to not compulsively pursue one medical educational opportunity after another. I'd rather live a shorter but more fulfilling life, than be old and miserable. I don't want to look back and say, "Well, it wasn't much fun, but I sure was around for a long time."

   Once one has done what is reasonable and appropriate with regard to health, it's time to move on to enjoying life. Don't let excessive anxiety over health ruin your participation in life.

10. *Write a brief description of what you want your life to mean—and think of it for a few minutes each day.* When you understand what life means to you, a lot of difficult health care problems get answered in the process.

11. *Memorize the "Four Steps to Better Care."* This should be familiar to you by now. You can understand not only

how the health care system operates, but can have a reasonable understanding of your own problems. You should be involved in your care as much as possible. The ultimate responsibility for your health is not with your physician but with yourself. You have an obligation to yourself and your family to act in the best interest of your care and their care. Accompanying this responsibility is the authority to decline recommendations if this is indicated, and take the initiative of looking at options that you feel best meet your own personal and particular needs. But, if you're going to decline, do it from a position of being well-informed and well-advised.

12. *Take to heart the rallying cry of the patient-consumer: Involve me! It's my health.* Let the medical people you are working with know that you *want* to be involved in your care. When you go to the hospital or the doctor's office, keep in mind that you have power.

. . .

This list isn't all-inclusive by any means. Be creative. See what else you can come up with that may be particularly applicable to your situation. In a very real way, just about all the recommendations of this book flow from full and active patient participation.

See if you can set aside a day specifically to accomplish these steps—they are at least as important as taking a day to clean out the garage or work in the yard. Your efforts will give you the foundation to start implementing "the fundamentals of long-term survival" to be discussed in the next chapter. These fundamentals are ongoing approaches to your health care rather than the more time limited efforts suggested here.

CHAPTER 24

The Ten Fundamentals of Long-Term Survival

Pearl:
If you want to live a long life, first have long-lived parents—then, make health care an important part of your existence.

Can people really increase their life spans?

There is a somewhat nihilistic approach to health care which might be called the "So Many Ticks Theory." It's talked about partly in jest and partly in earnest. It states that each of us are endowed at conception with our own particular number of heartbeats. When they are all used up—in our 40s, or 50s, or 60s, or whenever—then that's it. Period. Finito. Dead.

There is a kernel of truth in this theory that can't be ignored. I think that each of our bodies are genetically programmed to provide a life span within a limited range: One person is more likely to live to be 50, but not 70. Another person will live to be 80, but not 95. This, of course, assumes a "natural" death with no intervening occurrences such as succumbing to acute infections, accidents, or medical misadventures.

. . .

I believe that the ways to get all the "ticks" we're due fall into six general categories. Some examples are also included below.

- Avoid preventable illnesses: this would include such important contributors to a long life as getting immunizations, practicing good nutrition, not smoking, and avoiding liver disease from alcoholism, to name just a few.

- Prevent avoidable accidents: don't drink while driving, do wear protective gear for sports, don't leave guns and medications laying around at home, and do practice good safety habits on the job for example.

- Practice early disease detection: this would include such routine procedures as pap smears, mammograms, and regular blood pressure checks.

- Delaying the onset of poor health: you can avoid abusing your musculo-skeletal system and start watching your calorie intake.

- Get adequate treatment for chronic problems: this includes proper monitoring of medication, the use of regularly scheduled follow-up visits, and appropriate laboratory testing.

- Pay proper attention to new problems: be alert to new symptoms that develop (e.g., a significant change in bowel movements, or chest pain), and get prompt attention.

I'd estimate that—on average—Americans could add a decade or two to their life spans by following these simple steps. "Average" is the operant word here. If a motorcyclist who otherwise would have died at 40 due to a head injury starts wearing a helmet and lives to be 70, the average goes up a bit.

. . .

Here's my list of the ten most fundamental approaches I can suggest to increase one's chances for long term survival:

1. Establish a close, collaborative relationship with a doctor who will listen to you.
2. Use a hospital which is responsive to you.
3. Make health care education an important and regular part of your life.
4. Understand your illnesses and your medications as well as you can.
5. Keep your own set of regularly updated health records.
6. When treatment is suggested, look for options and consider all reasonable alternatives.
7. Get independent second opinions on major issues—both surgical and non-surgical.
8. Don't assume that health care providers are always correct (or even necessarily acting in your best interest).
9. Live a healthy and sane lifestyle.
10. Follow the "Four Steps to Better Care:" understanding, involvement, authority, responsibility.

. . .

I'll discuss each of these ten briefly:

1. While there is much more to good health care than having a doctor who will listen to you, this certainly is a major step in the right direction. A physician who listens will be in a much better position to make an accurate diagnosis upon which all further decisions can be based. And I think a doctor who will listen is more likely to be a doctor who will also be interested in you as a person, help you look at the best alternatives, and monitor your progress carefully. Additionally, a *healing* relationship can develop from a collaboration effort based on mutual respect, honesty, and caring.

2. Your choice of hospital may be somewhat limited due to insurance considerations, clinical resources, or your physician's practice or preference. Under the best of circumstances, hospital stays can be very difficult. A hospital which is patient-oriented can make the stay less of a problem (would "more pleasant" be too optimistic?), and even more survivable. Try to seek out an institution where patients are treated with respect and dignity. Ask your friends about their experiences.

3. In addition to our work and families, most of us have other aspects of our lives which are very important to us: sports, hobbies, music, theater, education, and religion, for example. How many of us would also make a similar commitment of time, money, and energy to include the assimilation of health care information? Would you routinely read about health care? Would you regularly watch and listen to educational programs on health presented on TV and radio? Take classes? Go to seminars? You should.

4. A significant part of your own health history involves your illnesses and your medications. If you have diabetes, high blood pressure, or any other chronic illness, you should know as much about them as you reasonably can. Occasionally, patients wind up knowing more than their doctors about a specific issue! If you are taking medications, you should know their intended use, possible side effects, potential interactions with other medications, and other significant aspects.

5. I have suggested that you request your medical records. This is only a start. Your health care may be provided by a number of people in a number of different settings. You may get some immunizations at a clinic, receive emergency care at an out-of-town hospital, and have your eyes tested by an optometrist in solo practice. You should be the one ultimately responsible for being sure that you have a complete set of these records. Any time you are hospitalized, request a discharge summary and add this to your collection. If you have surgery, request a copy of the operative report as well as the pathologist's report if tissue was removed.

   Now it's only fair to say that this isn't the way things are usually done. You'll be swimming upstream if you try. But I think it's the way it should be. Do the best you can.

6. There is often more than one way to treat a problem. If your physician does not volunteer options or alternatives, then ask about them. Even if several choices are forthcoming, you can still do your own research. I strive for the most conservative approach consistent with good medical practice. Also, see point number seven, below.

7. Major health care problems, in my mind, always warrant the consideration of an independent second opinion. I say "independent" because physicians will often refer their patients to like-minded colleagues. There's a rule in medicine that you don't send patients to your enemies. A doctor's referral to a close colleague may result in you getting a less useful consultation. There may simply be a lukewarm endorsement of a friend's recommendation. Patients may not recognize the potential harm in such an encounter.

   Second opinions shouldn't be confined only to the issue of surgical procedures. Other major health care problems may be equally benefited by a second opinion, especially if the course of the illness is not running smoothly.

8. Even in less critical circumstances than the major problems alluded to above, don't assume that health care workers always give the correct information. This point is my medical version of "let the buyer beware." Of course, don't assume that they're giving you incorrect information or bad advice either!

   Physicians and other caregivers can be victims of their own myths, haste, misinformation, and training. While you'll usually get reasonable information, you shouldn't feel reluctant to take the initiative in doing your own research. For instance, when a psychiatrist says you have a "chemical imbalance" that is causing your depression, how likely is this information to be correct? (Clue: The extent to which biology contributes to many mental illnesses is a hotly debated topic in psychiatry, but may not be presented to the patient as at all controversial or theoretical, but rather as fact.)

Hopefully, clinicians won't consciously work against your best interest. But they do have their own biases, prejudices, and perceived needs which won't necessarily serve you well. For instance, your operation may be scheduled based on your surgeon's vacation time rather than on your requirements. Or the hospital where the surgeon has privileges may not be the best equipped facility for the procedure in your area. And, other things being equal, surgeons will be inclined to recommend surgery and psychiatrists will be inclined to recommend formal mental health services—even when other options may serve you just as well.

9. Perhaps candles can be burned at both ends, but healthy lives can't. It's not difficult to learn about a healthy life-style. I think most people could generate a list of both good health habits and sane accident-prevention techniques (examples are given in the previous chapter). The trick, of course, is to *implement* what we know. It's that old devil "change"—a lot easier to say than to do. It can take resolve, support, energy, and effort. Efforts at change are often proportional to the seriousness of the consequences if you don't.

10. Today's patients should—perhaps, *must*!—feel empowered. It *is possible* for most people to understand how the health care system works. It *is possible* for them to understand issues concerning their own illnesses. This kind of knowledge can be used for maximum involvement in one's health care. Without that involvement, chances for success can be seriously diminished. Along with the authority of patients to make decisions (at least the decision to decline treatment or to search further), comes the responsibility

to do so wisely. Also there is the additional responsibility for living one's life in a reasonably healthy fashion.

Ideally, the patient will have developed a solid working relationship with a physician, and this can allow for more successful implementation of the "Four Steps to Better Care."

. . .

Health is a great deal more manageable than weather. Unlike the weather, we *can* do something about our health that may make decades of difference in our longevity. However, people need to realistically acknowledge their limitations in making improvements, as well as their potential to make a change for the better.

Some efforts are relatively easy, such as keeping an updated set of home health care records or subscribing to a health care magazine or newsletter. Other efforts are more difficult, such as living a healthy life style or changing bad habits.

You may choose to reject the more difficult efforts. You may choose to delegate your health care to physicians, hospitals, and others, who haven't the same vested interest in your life and happiness as you do. Regardless of how good their intentions and training, no one usually influences your health as much as you do. In a very important sense, you must be your own best doctor. Remember, doctor means "teacher." Teach yourself as much as you can about yourself!

CHAPTER 25

Quality Care for Everyone?

Pearl:

Unless patients have a greater involvement in their care (including financial decision-making), widely available quality care will remain outside our grasp.

Just as a child might turn his or her gaze away from a badly scraped knee, our nation has avoided carefully looking at the deep wounds of our health care system.

An honest look at the situation might be too distressing. It would require a painful examination of questionable professional standards and ethics, of declining personal values and responsibilities, and of our shaky philosophical underpinnings as a nation. We would have to acknowledge the limits and failings of medical science. We would discover that the greatest obstacle to better care is not overly expensive technology or even terrible disease. Instead, it is our own troubled psyches.

But we really must endure the pain of inspection. To start, we need a measuring stick. What are the very basic elements which *should* be contained within a quality health care delivery system? I propose the following:

- Physicians and other providers who are caring, competent, ethical, and professional in all ways.
- Patients who are informed, responsible, and involved—including having a very personal stake in the control of costs.
- A body of knowledge developed with intellectual honesty, leading to clinical accuracy and technological advancement.
- An infrastructure (hospitals, professional schools, equipment, clinics, a patient transport system, and so on) which is adequate to the task and whose parts are totally integrated with each other.
- An accessible system providing both value and equal quality for all, irrespective of any particular method of payment.
- An attitude that views health care more as a cherished national treasure—an honorable service of mutual participation rather than as a marketable commodity.

Is it really possible for everyone in this country receive such quality health care? This question is complex to say the least. The role of physicians is pivotal to any answer since tradition and reality have assigned them the major responsibility for health care in our society.

The obligations of physicians are essentially two-fold: (1) to professionally serve each patient to the highest standards, and (2) to provide leadership in accomplishing the six points listed above. Part of this second role is to be symbols of society's commitment to the high regard with which we hold human life.

I'm old-fashioned enough to think that words like "character," "morality," "responsibility," and "values" are more than rhetoric. Despite the fact that our society is adrift, it's still necessary for physicians, patients, or anyone else, to be measured against these terms. In fact, I suggest that the six points just listed could simply be summarized by the phrase "shared, morally-based health care," or "ShareMorCare" for short. I think this captures the essence of a participatory, value-based system of health care. With such an *attitude* we may not even need very much of a *plan* to revamp our system.

How do we currently measure up to the six basic points of a quality system? The report card is mixed with too many B's and C's and not enough A's. Since many of the troublesome elements have been discussed at length in earlier chapters, I'll only comment on a few of the more pertinent aspects here.

. . .

Patients and caregivers share many of the same strengths and failings. It's their strengths of bonding with others, creativity, sense of purpose, capacity for excellence, striving for knowledge, ability to act selflessly, and other positive human qualities that could drive a superb system of health care.

On the other hand, to whatever extent they have a narrowness of focus (territoriality), sense of emptiness, perception of unnecessary limitations, lack of foresight, self-absorption, and other potentially harmful characteristics; they stand in their own way on the road to better care.

But patients and caregivers can also be very different. Caregivers—who generally start out idealistically—often are beaten down by both self-inflicted wounds resulting from their own psycho-philosophies as well as by an inefficient and uncaring system. During years of training and practice, they incorporate within themselves the attitudes of the enveloping society. Physicians, especially, often develop an arrogance which compromises them individually and corrupts their profession as a whole.

Patients—and I'm speaking very generally—simply want what they can't have: Relief of all suffering, assurance of flawless care with little personal involvement, and a sustainable fantasy that death (which is almost always seen as bad) is avoidable. This attitude is conveyed as, "I have a problem—now, what are you going to do about it?"

Those involved directly in health care (patients, caregivers, and other members of the Biz-Med Complex) would benefit from an attitude that they are all participating in a personal and sacred service. The more health care is treated as a commodity, the more the foundation of a healing relationship is destroyed. The square pegs of commodities fit poorly into the round holes of the personal service concept of health care. To add to the problem, many of the round holes of the various parts of the health care system seem to be of different diameters, making service and cooperation within an integrated system almost impossible.

All of these problems work against the creation of quality health care that is available to everyone. But there are steps we can take to improve the situation. First, our society, to which health care is inexorably linked, can change. As long as we have hope, life, and free will; we can fulfill our potential as caring human beings. While keeping our freedom and capitalism, we can refocus on other basic ingredients: kindness, sharing, a pervading concern for our community and environment, personal understanding of clinical and delivery issues, and a constant striving for improvement. All these are significant elements of successful health care. If I sound like a Pollyanna, I won't apologize. Without these attitudes, forget about our system even approaching the desired ideal.

Within the health care community, the patient—not the administrator, third-party payer, bureaucrat, or even the caregiver—should be the most central figure. Ultimately, the delivery of service becomes an interaction between one individual healer and the one who requires healing. Both have tremendous responsibilities.

If either party is more responsible, it would be the caregivers. Healing is their special area of training, what they get paid to do, what they have dedicated themselves to do. It is they who should control much of the structure and infrastructure of the Biz-Med Complex. They must accept the *major* responsibility.

While a patient's responsibility is also large, he or she may be too ill to exercise it when the need is greatest. And certainly the individual's general level of medical knowledge cannot reasonably be expected to match that of the professionals. Still, the patient holds the *ultimate* responsibility for his or her personal health care.

Caregivers need to re-dedicate themselves in a world which is more and more devoid of commitment and professionalism. They can develop more health care-related educational opportunities and facilities in their communities. These, in turn, can help produce greater numbers of qualified health care professionals—even if this means less money for each individual caregiver who is trained.

These additional practitioners, responding in part to economic and personal factors, would redistribute themselves to rural and inner-city areas. If further impetus to relocation was necessary, such service could become a precondition of admission to schools which are financed by public funds.

We can teach these practitioners more efficiently, and we can also teach them to practice in markedly more efficient ways, to be aware of the suffering and needs of those whom they serve. The privilege to serve must be emphasized. We can start the process of developing better caregivers by admitting more well-rounded and dedicated individuals to medical schools and other professional training facilities. Many nurses could better serve by becoming physicians via innovative programs rather than by becoming nurse-practitioners.

Patients can make their own significant contributions. Health care information and healthy practices can become as much of their lives as are clothes, sports, hobbies, cars—even jobs. They can take it upon themselves to be knowledgeable and prudent with regard to their own health and that of their families. They can develop their own basic at-home health care libraries.

Empowerment of patients will help give them an equal—but different—role on the health care team. They can bring a reasonable "civilian" level of understanding to health care issues. They can be assertive and inquisitive, while doing their part to foster an atmosphere of cooperation, mutual respect, and understanding. If the patient role extends to direct financial involvement in the cost of their care, all the better. The crowning achievement would be when patients not only become participants in their care, but work *collaboratively* with their caregivers.

. . .

What are some of the options we have for building a better health care system? These options can be divided into two groups: those concerned with the actual delivery of care, and those concerned with paying for the cost of that interaction.

With regard to delivery of care, we could:

- Rely on via managed care with its emphasis on cost-effectiveness
- Wait for the development of a higher standard of professionalism within the entire Biz-Med Complex
- Encourage patients to gain greater understanding and involvement and exercise their responsibility and authority
- Change nothing, but hope for the best
- Implement a combination of some of the above

With regard to payment, here are some of the options:

- Employers pay more (all?) of the cost
- The government assumes more or all of the cost via an increasing array of various entitlement programs
- The government makes the funds available, but the patients decide (with appropriate provider input) how to spend them
- If we can achieve full employment, everyone buys private insurance or pays cash
- Change nothing, but hope for the best
- Implement a combination of some of the above

The primary concern should be how (and consequently, at what level of quality) care is delivered at the patient-provider level. The mechanism of payment, while *extremely* important, is still secondary.

From the possible options given in the two lists above, what's best in the long run? If there were a simple answer to this, our country probably wouldn't be in its current dilemma over health care. But complexity doesn't mean that common sense can't prevail.

Here's the answer which I feel reflects common sense and my experience: Encourage the "professionals" to live up to their name. Students who start out wanting to be their own particular profession's "Marcus Welbys" should be supported in that effort, not impeded. Patients can no longer sit back and "let doc do it" or "let the government do it." The potential for healthier life, as well as the responsibility and authority to realize that potential is within the grasp of most individuals. We can insist that the entire Biz-Med Complex fulfills its mission in an integrated and caring fashion.

Finally, put the purse-strings in the patients' hands—thereby letting millions upon millions of potential health care "mini-experts" decide how they want their dollars spent.

All these features could come together within the context of a culture of healing—and be honored as such by our nation. But how does each patient—rich or poor—get an opportunity for equitable financial involvement in his or her own health care?

. . .

Here's a scenario I'll put forth as a possible plan. Look at it as a starting point—some food for thought. It has some of the elements which have been described in the media (along with other payment schemes) as a "medical savings account." Because of its more hands-on approach, I'd describe my plan more as "money under the mattress" than as a "savings account."

Start with an agency establishing a simple system of a 1 to 10 scale of the health risks for individuals based on only age and formal diagnoses: A "1" would be someone who is young and healthy. A "10" would be an older person with many known chronic health problems. Everyone else would be somewhere in between. And everyone would be given an account with an assigned dollar amount to use. This system would have to be worked out in an initial cooperative effort between government, professionals, academics, consumers, and the business community (including the Biz-Med Complex). But the formula for its application to individuals should be straightforward.

The total amount of all the assignments nationwide would equal only what we are currently spending on health care, which is probably about $4,000 per person. Everyone would share proportionately based on their place on the scale. No "new" money would be involved. On a yearly basis, everyone's assignment would be placed in their "health care account" at the insurance carrier of their choice. The companies would agree to accept everyone for the assignment specified on their scale of 1 to 10. Then people could draw from their own accounts for all of their health care expenses: doctors, hospitals, prescriptions, dentists, glasses, testing. *Everything.*

Individuals could pick any insurance company they wished as their agent to receive and disperse the funds. At the end of the year, anything remaining in the account, minus a small management fee to the insurance company, would be split between the individual and the government. (Some mechanism might need to be provided to prevent individuals from being inappropriately stingy in getting care, especially when children were involved.) The government's half would go to a "super fund" to help back up the insurers for overdrawn accounts. Families with few problems and/or careful management could receive significant refunds. If one believes that there's even a modicum of truth in the saying that "the seat of the psyche is in the wallet," there would probably be little, if any spending over current levels on a nationwide basis, even with an increase in offered benefits. People would quickly learn to seek value for their medical dollar.

This could be done without much dislocation of the traditional structure of our present system. Insurance companies would have a somewhat different role, but could still compete for business based on their own efficiencies, images, lower management fees, educational efforts, other assistance to their clients, and customer satisfaction. The better the company you select, the more funds you would be likely to have left at the end of the year.

Insurance companies would offer only *one* level of coverage: Virtually *everything* that an involved, responsible patient and an ethical, competent physician considered reasonable. They would, of course, first look at the risks and benefits of that care. If necessary, companies could apply to the "super fund" for reimbursement in the event of a deficit year or to cover certain individuals with extremely high medical expenses.

In this way, all people would be covered equally for extensive services. And if it were more expensive, is that a disaster?

What we really want is *value* for our health care dollar, not cheap health care.

Perhaps the expense of care would skyrocket. In a worst case scenario, we could then have a national referendum to determine a "cap" to the upper limit of spending, and recognize that some services would no longer be available to anyone. Then and only then would we have "rationing." But citizens must be making these decisions, not a faceless bureaucracy.

For the sake of space, this plan is presented in fairly broad strokes. Careful readers will understand that significant aspects are not presented here.

Whether or not health care is a right is, for me, immaterial to this discussion. I don't know about you, but I wouldn't want to be part of a society where we didn't have the level playing field of equal quality care for all. I wouldn't want access to life-saving surgery which was denied for purely financial reasons to my neighbor.

. . .

In addition to the measures already described, a great many other efforts could keep costs down. Hospitals and doctors could follow sound business and management practices to become more efficient. Care could be kept simple, but effective. With well-implemented preventative programs, careful history-taking leading to accurate diagnosis, good clinical record-keeping, sticking to essential treatment regimens without all the trimmings, and using mid-level practitioners where appropriate, costs could be significantly reduced.

There should be a level of professional fees that are commensurate with a doctor's education, but not the outlandish ones currently found. Patients and doctors should learn to work—and save money—together. Finally, we'd need a way of sensibly and adequately compensating patients who have adverse clinical results, without the extravagance of a runaway tort system which functions more as a big bucks lottery.

An objection to this overall approach might be that we can't afford either present or future technological advances. I see the answer to this concern as having four components: (1) as a truly caring society, we need to re-think the ethics of desperate, "heroic" care which often hurts more than helps, (2) our demonstrated entrepreneurial spirit will help bring down costs for those technologies which are truly beneficial (similar to what happened to the cost of computers and fax machines), (3) savings could come from the patient-controlled funding process I described, as well as a participatory or even fully collaborative relationship between patient and doctor, and (4) cures will come—and once discovered will have no further research costs associated with them.

. . .

Could these proposed changes to care ever work? I certainly hope so. Harnessing our innate positive values, we could look forward optimistically. Otherwise, our health care delivery system will be condemned to patchwork care. And we may be condemned to having just the mere appearance of being a caring people.

Ideas in this chapter have attempted to emphasize the central position of the patient in any system; the importance of monetary control by the patient; and the unique (and irreplaceable) role of the physician, especially, but other caregivers as well. The practice of medicine is kept as the province of the physician, while financial and personal decisions are properly assigned to the patient. The manner in which patients would respond collectively to such a system would say a great deal about ourselves as a society. The same could be said for the physicians' response.

If you don't like my ideas for change as expressed in this chapter, I challenge you to come up with something better. I'd be overjoyed if you did!

. . .

Perhaps some of the underlying ideas expressed in this chapter do sound like "pie in the sky" concepts. But they could work. After all, good care on an individual level essentially takes only a good doctor, a good patient who feels empowered, access to some reasonable and well-integrated resources, and a little efficiency—all in the context of a caring society with its priorities sorted out. We should be able to do that.

What won't work are efforts to legislate quality; to take the health care dollars out of the hands of the patients who are best able to control its use; and to turn over certain areas of care from the acknowledged expertise of specialists to well-meaning, but often ill-equipped generalists and others who may not be prepared to provide adequate quality of care. Even worse would be to give control to the bureaucrats.

CHAPTER 26

Finally Making Sense of the Chaos

Pearl:
Better care starts by respecting the patient who is at its center.

As individuals—and as a nation—we're sinking into a muddy, unstable ground of chaotic health care delivery. Rarely does our care reach its full potential; sometimes it's downright dangerous.

How ironic this is! Society has set the medical world apart so that it could contain and tame some of our worst fears: pain, suffering, infirmity, hopelessness, isolation, loss, madness, the unknown and—ultimately—death itself. We worship its practitioners and bestow offerings upon this modern religion in the hope that it will ward off the demons that threaten to expose our vulnerabilities. Yet too often it turns on us with malevolence. As broken as the system of health care delivery may be, it is still fixable.

Even when it is not seriously injurious to the patient, the health care system can suffer from being inefficient and ineffective. Care is frequently devoid of both compassion from the caregivers and participation—much less collaboration—by the patient. Costs seem out of control. Public dissatisfaction is high.

What went wrong? Fingers are often pointed at failings which are largely economic, technological, political, demographic, or regulatory in nature. These *are* problems. But they are not the root causes. For the basic problem, it's necessary to understand the people and organizations involved in care—especially patients, doctors, and hospitals. "Soft" issues are prominent here—the kind without much glamour, the kind which would make for poor sound bites and poor visual imagery on the evening news. They wouldn't fit easily into political platforms; they are nevertheless critical issues.

These problems relate to the perceptions and forces which influence health care delivery, as well as to reality:

1. Lack of philosophy. If we lack a bedrock foundation of meaning and purpose in our lives, we'll have no rudder or compass for navigating health care delivery issues. This philosophical omission leaves inadequately answered such pertinent questions as: "What is the meaning of life? What is the purpose of health care? Who is really responsible for that care?"

2. Lack of understanding. The system of care, the people involved, and the basic scientific and clinical issues are inherently complex. Familiarity on at least a minimum level provides the tools to build a better system. This process starts with parents. They need to teach their children that health—like morals, education, or money management—is important. Schools must continue this process by providing better education and the example of teachers as role models.

3. Lack of approaches. Like a plane approaching a nearly weathered-in airport, health care needs a plan to reach its goal during the current turbulence. The aircraft may

be functioning perfectly, but the pilot still needs his instructions. The lack of practical methods or procedures for an integrated delivery of care is a major cause of our current chaos. We need a plan for professionals and patients alike.

4. Lack of empowerment. Patients often feel too overwhelmed by—and left out of—a complicated process and an arcane body of knowledge. They don't see how to participate in the system in a meaningful way. Surprisingly, physicians also can have a sense of isolation and powerlessness in attempting to implement productive change.

5. Lack of a unifying thread. The fabric of health care has unraveled. It could make a marvelous garment if it could only be held together in an organized and comprehensible fashion.

It should be obvious that there's no necessity to point fingers at just the professionals or just the patients. There's plenty of blame for everyone. But even more important, there's plenty of *opportunity* for all.

. . .

Many of the deficits described in the above points could be summarized by saying that our society lacks a culture of healing. How did these defects come to be? In part, they resulted from some tough ingredients being blended into an unpalatable stew. For physicians, these ingredients are a body of knowledge which is complex, training which is often inadequate and arduous (and often demeaning), professionalism which is demanding, and tasks which are often unpleasant.

For patients, there is the understandable distaste of dealing with their own mortality and frailties. And not everyone wishes to be well-informed about a profession which passes its days opening up abdomens, dissecting the dead, controlling the psychotic, delivering the newborn, and presiding over the last moments of life.

Largely by the default of others, physicians have acquired much of the power. But they aren't necessarily best-suited for the task. Now the profession helps direct medicine as it goes far beyond its appropriate boundaries. Yet, in other ways, physicians seem inadequate to carrying out their true responsibilities.

The chaos is worsened because we are a society mired in a multitude of almost unsolvable social problems. The "caring" professions have not been immune to society's greed, materialism, and generally unsatisfying search for meaning. In addition, society and professionals have been unable to provide either vision or leadership—in part because they cannot end their marriage to unworkable but cherished beliefs in a paternalistic system which largely excludes patients from involvement in their own care.

. . .

Given the current turmoil in health care, can a productive response be made by individuals, the Biz-Med Complex, or by our nation? The short answer is an emphatic, "Yes!"

Both patients and caregivers are capable of articulating a clearer philosophy. Almost everyone can develop a concept of who they are, how they fit into the world, their importance to each other, and the role of a healthy life and a good death within these contexts.

Physicians and patients can understand each other's needs and perspectives. The more that physicians can come to know their own humanity and vulnerabilities, the more they can therapeutically touch the needs of their patients. They can teach patients how to work more effectively with the professionals. Patients can make acquiring health care information a priority in their lives. And patients can even help their caregivers to do better jobs. After all, we physicians are fond of saying that, "We learn from our patients."

By using the "Four Steps to Better Care," patients and caregivers can weave themselves into the larger system. Financially, patients should get involved in the dollar consequences of their care. The more involvement they have monetarily, the less the care is likely to cost.

People who are able to *understand* how health care is delivered will likely get better care than those who lack this knowledge. Those who are actively *involved*—and even better, those who are working collaboratively with their physicians—are positioned to get better care than who sit passively at the mercy of the system. Those who exercise their *authority* over their own care, while balancing it with their *responsibility* to see to their own health, can also fare better than those who simply relinquish those rights to others.

Patients, caregivers and others within the Biz-Med Complex all need empowerment to achieve their maximum effectiveness. Working together, they could position the patient in the appropriate spot: at the very center of the health care world.

Increased professionalism is an important thread that can tie together better health care. But perhaps the single most important thread would be a global mission statement by the Biz-Med Complex which states the Complex's commitment to developing an integrated system of service to patients, in addition to meeting its financial goals. This could lead to what is truly shared, morally-based health care—ShareMorCare.

The old covenant between patient and doctor (captured in part by the phrase "trust me, I'm a doctor") is neither workable or maximally beneficial. A new covenant of mutual respect and participation—a collaborative practice, if you will—can bring more satisfying results to both patient and doctor.

. . .

But patients and doctors don't exist in isolation from the larger society. People and society change each other—for better or for worse—in their interactions.

Society can also provide part of the solution for better care by understanding that its role in the cure for our unhealthy system is not primarily financial: It is largely one of attitude. Its major role is in providing the stable, supportive, caring "culture" upon which quality, access, and affordability can all be adequately implemented.

Whether or not you see our nation as moving into a new era of more satisfying health services largely depends on your optimism or pessimism regarding our society as a whole. If you're optimistic, you see the essential elements of an effective health care system as being obtainable. You believe that we have the national gumption to cure our health care wounds as a society. You see the crucial players as responsible individuals who are held accountable for their actions—be they patients or caregivers.

There is a saying to the effect that "what is honored in a country will be practiced there." If we honor the virtues and characteristics implicit in a caring society and a caring profession, then caring will be practiced without being legislated (as if it *could* be legislated).

If you are pessimistic and see little hope for basic change from within our society, then you'll be forced by default to rely heavily on legislation and regulation. This would represent an effort to simultaneously "cut our losses" financially while still appearing to care despite all evidence to the contrary. This is denial on a national scale—but a defense mechanism of which we are quite capable.

. . .

Currently, our system seems trapped in mediocrity. Most people have some entitlement to benefits, but no guarantee of real "care." At best, improvement will take time—there are no quick fixes. Professionals will ultimately deliver to people the level of care—good or bad—which society implicitly requests of them. In a very real sense, society is the ultimate arbitrator of care, even being capable of overriding the efforts of a powerful profession.

The task of delivering high quality, accessible care is worth the effort for all parties involved. The world of health care already can provide much of what is of critical value and great comfort to the patient. But so much more is possible. Professionals would do well to start to acknowledge their limitations, while better utilizing their talents and resources.

A major step for moving ahead is to emphasize prevention, while more broadly defining this concept. The health care system needs to encourage not only traditional preventive measures such as immunizations, but also safer environments, greater personal security, a more premeditated approach to decision-making in treatment issues, more time for people to devote to health-promoting efforts, and the promulgation of a culture of healing without crossing the line to a cult of healing. That is, it's time for us to stop shooting ourselves in the foot and then trying to repair the damage. Let's just not pull the trigger in the first place.

Putting physicians back in charge of the practice of medicine, and patients in charge of financial decisions, would also be positive steps. The federal government may have a significant role as a facilitator and leader, but it is incapable of being a "national physician."

We also need to adjust our mindset regarding suffering and death. The avoidance of these are not the absolute goals of health care. We need to clearly define our health care goals as a society if we hope to achieve them.

To reach our health care goals, we'll have to harness our most valuable untapped medical resource:

> *People*—Their potential to understand how care is delivered, and to use that knowledge productively.

Then we can usher in a new era of care even more revolutionary than has been brought by modern technology itself!

APPENDIX A

More of Understanding People and Organizations

In Chapter Two, I made an effort to provide a framework for understanding health care's two basic components: People and organizations. The people include (1) patients and (2) all those involved within the Biz-Med Complex, especially practitioners. The organizations include professional groups such as the AMA, institutions such as hospitals and clinics, and many others.

This effort was made to allow the reader to move from a knowledge based primarily on "facts" (cost, number of doctors and hospitals, results of surveys, and so on) to a knowledge based at the level of *how* and *why* health care functions as it does.

My position is that this latter, more fundamental level of understanding has been ignored for too long in health care. Such a history of avoidance is in part due to the belief that ordinary people couldn't understand anything so complex. The prevailing attitude was "leave it to the professionals." With today's more educated and informed public, that's not necessary. Most people could now have the kind of knowledge which allows fuller, more productive participation in their care—and for better decision-making at the health care policy level.

No one is the sole proprietor of the absolute truth when it comes to conceptualizing health care. Certainly, I'm not. But to aid understanding I have used two approaches which I find both useful and reasonably simple. These involve people's *perceptions* on the one hand and the *forces* acting upon individuals and organizations on the other. These significant influences are, of course, in addition to the obvious impact of *reality* itself—and the ability of people to still make a free choice.

In essence, I maintain that perceptions and forces—and their cumulative effects upon us over the years—have been given inadequate attention. While it's true that these influences may be subtle and not easily recognizable, their impact can be tremendous.

For the interested reader—those who like their theories on the esoteric side—I promised in Chapter Two an "advanced course" of such an understanding. So, in this appendix I'll be presenting a somewhat more detailed exposition of these perceptions and forces. There's no claim that this material represents any great discovery by me—or even that it will withstand the test of time intact as presented here. I consider it a "work in progress." In fact, I change it frequently. But, in this Appendix, concepts are presented as I currently see them. Your lists of forces and perceptions might differ somewhat from mine. A summary diagram (Figure 3) will aid you in putting it all together.

While the two models to be described do have some overlap, I've separated them from each other the best I could. For example, the *purpose* we see in our lives comes largely from our perceptions. But, at the same time, the *purpose* for which we live acts as a force upon us.

The focus of the "Spectrum of Human Concerns" is on perceptions. I see it as looking at our lives primarily from intellectual and philosophical viewpoints. An accompanying chart (Figure 4) lists eleven core issues or concerns and their ranges.

Each issue has a positive (+) and a negative (-) pole. For example, relationships are a core issue of concern to us all. They range from solid social bonding at one pole to feelings of extreme isolation at the other. Similarly, our involvement with life itself ranges from tight control to an accepting passivity.

The focus of GHIDS (Group Hypothetical Inertial Directives) and PHIDS (Personal Hypothetical Inertial Directives) is more psychologically oriented. (Both rhyme with "kids" and are pronounced "gids" and "fids.") These are forces which may come either from within or arise externally; they drive or motivate (i.e., they give directives). GHIDS affect groups; PHIDS affect individual people.

Simply put, they represent possible explanations (hypotheses) for why groups and individuals either change or remain the same (i.e., have inertia). A list of PHIDS and GHIDS is shown in Figures 5 and 6. The GHIDS are relatively self-explanatory. So are most of the PHIDS; in this "advanced," but still brief presentation, I've elected to rely on the reader's ingenuity to elucidate those meanings which are not immediately apparent.

The basic lesson here is that decisions and behaviors are not always explainable simply by what is observable on the surface. The Spectrum of Human Concerns and the GHIDS/PHIDS can be useful tools for understanding what occurs below the surface. Such information can ultimately be more important than the mere facts and figures; it can help patients get better care, help policy makers formulate better plans, and help us all understand more fully about our health care organizations. A knowledge of these influences can help us in non-clinical areas of life as well.

Reaching for such enlightened goals of understanding may sound a little grandiose. So, I suggest you evaluate these approaches based on your own insights, experiences, and instincts. Use what you can, or modify them so that they can work for you. I think you'll find them to be useful, though still imperfect, tools for your understanding of people and organizations in general. And, when applied to health care, they can help you make greater sense out of the apparent chaos.

Psycho-Philosophical Factors✤ Influencing Care
Figure 3

Type	Label	Definition
PERCEPTIONS	Spectrum of Human Concerns	How we "see" life
FORCES	PHIDS	What motivates or drives us (or allows us to operate)
FORCES	GHIDS	What motivates or drives (or allows to operate)

✤Some factors overlap, e.g. "purpose" is both a force and a perception.

Nature	Involvement	Examples
Intellectual ✣✣ and Philosophical	People	• Bonding • Purpose • Ignorance • Chaos • Passivity • Control • Survival
Psychological	People (PHIDS)	• Self-Esteem • Fantasy • Money • "Territoriality" • Purpose • "Now-ness"
Psychological	Organizations (GHIDS)	• Functions more as a collection of individuals • "Bigger is better" • Have a stated mission, but will adapt to survive

✣✣ Even intellectual aspects are ultimately perceived philosophically.

The Spectrum of Human Concerns
Figure 4

Positive Pole (+)	Core Issues	Negative Pole (–)
Joy	Pleasure	Sadness
Order	Structure	Chaos
Bonding	Relationships	Isolation
Knowledge	Understanding	Ignorance
Survival	Existence	Mortality
Control	Involvement	Passivity
Perfection	Development	Limitations
Hope	Expectation	Despair
Purpose	Meaning	Emptiness
Clear	Reality	Obscure
Power	Strength	Weakness

Note: The designation of poles as positive and negative is some what arbitrary. For example, a "positive" such as control can be overdone, whereas a "negative" such as sadness canhave its own ultimate benefits.

PHIDS
Figure 5

Personal Hypothetical Inertial Directives

Money
Power
Control
Connectedness
Territoriality
Individuation
Compassion
Intimacy
Self-Esteem
Respect
Me-ness
Potential
Now-ness
Knowledge
Purpose
Fantasy
Happiness
Sexuality

Familiarity
Aggression
Religion
Growth
Survival
"Immortality"
Love
Excellence
Fairness
Altruism
"Psychological-Baggage"
Guilt
Accommodation
Hope
Fear
Creativity
Entitlement
Reason

GHIDS
Figure 6

Group Hypothetical Inertial Directives

1. Function more as collections of *individuals* than "en masse."
2. Collectively are "smarter" than individuals, but less flexible.
3. Frequently have a stated mission.
4. Exhibit more of a "focus" than a "mission" in day-to-day activity.
5. Have concerns, but no morals.
6. Highly value their existence—often taking uncharacteristic actions to survive.
7. Will even change their original mission in order to survive (i.e., they have lives of their own apart from their stated purpose).
8. Have a "collective power" greater than the sum of the power of the individuals.
9. Rarely have—or stick to—a pre-determined life-span.
10. Operate as if "more" and "bigger" were better, causing them to grow/acquire.
11. Act for reasons specific to themselves which may not be comprehensible outside the organizations.
12. Usually have the seat of their collective psyches located in their bookkeeping departments.
13. Function in a manner giving priority to their own convenience.
14. Can make idiotic mistakes in spite of polished images.
15. Have poor internal communications as one of their biggest foes.
16. Sometimes value the *appearance* of action more than its actual occurrence.

APPENDIX B

Brief Personal Medical History Form

Brief Personal Medical History Form

Name ______________________________

Date form completed ______________________

Primary physician ________________ Phone __________

Other physicians ________________ Phone __________

________________ Phone __________

Insurance carrier ________________ Phone __________

In emergency notify ________________ Phone __________

Current Medications

Name	Purpose	Dose	When First Started

Illnesses, injuries, and operations (Indicate with * if hospitalized)

Diagnosis	Year	Treatment	Results

Disabilities, if any

____

____

Allergies

Drug or Substance	Reaction	Treatment, if any

Special diet?

____

Where is "Living Will" kept? (or circle: None)

____

Where is "Durable Power of Attorney for Health Care" kept? (or circle: None)

____

Parents

	Age (or Age at Death)	Health Status (or Cause of Death)	Significant Illnesses
Mother			
Father			

Important examinations / Test results (e.g., complete physical, EKG)

Type	Data	Results

Weight _____ lbs. Blood pressure ___ / _____

Other pertinent information? ______________________________

To the reader: Photocopy this form after completing it. Keep copies in convenient places (your health care file, glove compartment, etc.)—but keep it private. Use the reverse side of the form for updates and additional information.

APPENDIX C

An Invitation For Readers To Respond

Dear Reader,

I hope you have found this book to be interesting, practical, and stimulating. Perhaps the material has brought to your mind some of your own experiences or thoughts regarding health care.

There are tentative plans to gather readers' input into a subsequent volume along with my comments. If you are interested in having your material considered for inclusion (after editing or abstracting, if necessary), please write me at: TLM Consulting, P.O. Box 293, Monticello, IL 61856. All contributor's identities will be protected in print. Please include in your letter the following statement: "Dr. Minogue has my permission to use this letter without compensation under the conditions indicated in Appendix C of "*Trust Me, I'm a Doctor*." On the front of the envelope, mark: ATTENTION: BOOK.

While the publication of such a follow-up book is not assured, I feel that a discussion of readers' responses to "*Trust Me, I'm a Doctor*" (whether in agreement or disagreement) could further the cause of better personal and national health care. I regret that individual responses will not be possible.

Very truly yours,

Thomas L. Minogue, M.D.

Thomas L. Minogue, M.D.

Dr. Minogue is on the faculty of the University of Illinois and is President of TLM Consulting, as well as being a licensed private pilot.